TAKING THE LEAD

LOUISE GIROUX

TAKING THE LEAD
DANCING WITH CHRONIC ILLNESS

Northstone

Editors: Michael Schwartzentruber, Dianne Greenslade
Cover design, artwork, and interior design: Margaret Kyle
Consulting art director: Robert MacDonald

We acknowledge the financial support of the Government of Canada through the Book Publishing Industry Development Program for our publishing activities.

Northstone Publishing Inc. is an employee-owned company, committed to caring for the environment and all creation. Northstone recycles, reuses and composts, and encourages readers to do the same. Resources are printed on recycled paper and more environmentally friendly groundwood papers (newsprint), whenever possible.
The trees used are replaced through donations to the Scoutrees For Canada Program.
Ten percent of all profit is donated to charitable organizations.

Canadian Cataloguing in Publication Data
Louise Giroux, 1951–
Taking the lead
Includes bibliographical references.
ISBN 1-896836-20-8
1. Chronic diseases – Psychological aspects. 2. Chronically ill – Psychology. I. Title
R726.5.G57 1998 155.9'16 C97-911088-2

Published by Northstone Publishing Inc.
Kelowna, British Columbia, Canada

Printing
9 8 7 6 5 4 3 2

Printed in Canada by Transcontinental Printing
Louiseville, Quebec

To my Heroes and Heroines, the professional dancers

and

to Dr. William McMullen, my physician

and

to Dr. Bernie Siegel, my mentor

The author welcomes letters from her readers.

Louise Giroux
Box 172, Station Q
Toronto, ON
M4T 2M1

CONTENTS

ACKNOWLEDGEMENTS

I would like to acknowledge the staff and the interns of The Pastoral Institute of Northern Ontario, especially Reverend Melvin Rose, Clinical Director and Ms. Marion Kennedy-MacQueen, Administrator, for their support in my quest toward holistic wellness.

A special "Thank You" to Monique Taylor, my dear friend and writing consultant; in appreciation for the manuscript editing and for her encouragement in revealing, through my writing, my true self.

INTRODUCTION

Would You Like to Dance?

I do not live with chronic illness. It lives with me.

For me, learning to live with chronic illness was like learning to dance with a very awkward partner (not to mention the awkward partner that I was myself). In the beginning, it was a hard struggle. Sometimes I slid, stumbled, or fell out of step. At other times, to my great amazement, I experienced myself as graceful as I met the every day, every second, challenge of chronic illness.

The metaphor of the dance is appropriate since it conjures up images of a partnership and although illness is never a wanted partner it establishes itself in our lives with or without our consent. Even more, I realize I need to *take the lead* in this partnership, this dance, if I am to use the power of my chronic illness to reshape my life in a more positive way. Taking the lead assures the empowerment of the person who lives with chronic illness and guarantees that they will never become their disease.

My story is not uncommon but rather the story of every man and woman who dances with illness. The story tells of life before the diagnosis, how the illness first manifested itself, the changes that it brought about and how I work diligently at living in rhythm with it.

Because the challenge of living with chronic illness is three dimensional – that is physical, emotional and spiritual – I need to deal on all three levels to achieve wellness. The physical challenge of a chronic illness is easiest to deal with; the symptoms are signals that one can attend to with medication and proper symptom management. However, the emotional challenge stretches our limits. We experience feelings of such a vast range and nature that we discover our feeling self as never before; it is as though chronic illness generates a myriad of feelings by which one can easily become one of the walking wounded, a bleeding creature of feeling. The spiritual challenge, perhaps because of its nebulous character, is often the last dimension we deal with. Yet paradoxically, the spirit is where lies solace, sense of purpose, and genuine peace and acceptance.

These are some of the facets of chronic illness that make it mandatory for the individual to develop a list of heroes, of champions, who have lived fully in spite of chronic illness; they have had a quality of life, which inspires and energizes the chronically challenged person. Holistic wellness is the perfect prescription for holistic challenge.

Throughout *Taking the Lead*, you will meet Leah, Bob, and Sarah. These three challenged persons will welcome you into their lives, their individual dances with chronic illness. As you come to know them and watch them as they negotiate with their dance partner, at times more effectively than others, you will gain a better understanding of some of the ways in which to take the lead with chronic illness.

Chronically ill persons and their caregivers face common challenges. All suffer from the illness, and all must learn to dance with it. In a way, either by diagnosis or by osmosis, all are affected. For this reason, all of the material in this book refers to both sides of the world of chronic illness.

So you never learned to dance? You've been told you have two left feet? Here is a new beginning for you. If you live facing the challenge of chronic illness in your life or in the life of someone you love, you have no choice but to master the dance. Once you put on your dancing shoes, find the proper music, create the appropriate atmosphere, *you will lead* your chronic illness, your partner, onto the dance floor like a world-champion dancer, with dignity and grace.

ONE

My Story

My Dance

Who am I?

Only in my mind do I dance
Only in my imagination do I walk
Only in my memory do I climb
As if who I am is not who I was.

For eternal hours I worry
For eternal seconds I glimpse at hope
For nights I sit and stare
As if I will never rebecome who I was.

When eyes pierce into mine I turn away
When voices speak tenderness I do not listen
When hands hold me I pull away
As if I am repulsed by who I have become.

Where did the energy of my soul disappear
Where did the music of my voice wander
Where did the sound of my footsteps go
As if I have lost who I was.

From My diary...

September 25, 1994

This morning I visited my past. I became aware last week that my courage and my acceptance had reached such a degree that for the first time since I left this high school, eight years ago, I actually wanted to go back for a visit.

From 1970 to 1986, for 15 years...In high-heeled shoes my feet and legs walked through the halls of this school. A typical work day ran from 7:30 in the morning until 5:00 in the afternoon, with way too much coffee in between. I taught the standard five days and taught two more days of extra-curricular activities. My energy level replenished itself swiftly, my cerebral juices flowed wildly, my emotions gauged themselves healthily and my spirit flourished towards fulfilment. I embraced my sense of purpose, my chosen profession, with love and zest.

From 1986 to 1994, 8 years... With dormant feet I stand on what feel like footballs. Walking is most awkward and at times impossible. My niece inherits my high-heeled shoes. I dance in my head. The rapid staccato of those shoes in the corridors of the school echoes in my memory; sunshine images linger in my mind's eye of walking a 25-kilometer marathon with my students. In the darkness, at a snail's pace, I crawl during the long hours of my insomniac nights.

Most days I celebrate scheduled mild activity. I replenish that frail energy with frequent naps during the day. At times, to my terror, my thinking is blurred, I forget things, I am confused and even too weak to think or to speak. I ride an emotional roller coaster which traps me in loops of anger and rage. I meditate daily, even when I feel only a void. I pray, I listen, I reflect and gradually a light sparks; the flames dance within the fire of my soul.

Who am I?
What do I contribute to the world as I lie in my bed?
Who pulled the plug on my life?
Maybe I died and they forgot to bury me.

Around 9:00 in the morning, I park in front of the school. There have been drastic changes here. The tiny bushes we pioneers planted 20 years ago are now mature cedars but the red storage shed still stands. I stare at the red brick. Everything is so familiar. But the old has been recycled into new.

I wait for Mel to take out my scooter as butterflies flutter in my stomach. Two years of repeated invitation have been turned down. How I have wanted to be able to come here today, to attain the emotional strength, to feel safe emotionally to visit. It is time for me. It feels right.

Since my last acute relapse, my feet are numb and I drag my left leg; I can barely walk. As I hear the motor of my scooter run smoothly, I register this sound, so different from my high heels hitting the terrazzo floor.

Freedom, I think. These wheels bring freedom and independence.

My dear old friend, now the principal, greets me with eye contact that seems to scream, "So happy to see you here, I have been waiting for you." My eyes are not deceiving me, I hope. I catch sight of Ann, running toward me with open arms. This is recycling in its pure form. I wonder if while she teaches, she sits in the seat where I used to teach her? Serge, the newest addition to the social science department calls us to the staff room: "Just like you, Madame, I teach history, but I'm not as much fun as you were!" It is Pauline's animated face that appears around the corner. "I knew I would cry when I saw you; I guess it's because I'm a teacher because of you." Over coffee, I laugh boisterously and I hold back tears...this is so touching; there are six teachers here who were my students years ago. I loved them passionately when they were 15, I love them passionately now when they are 30.

Michel is radiant this morning. "You have risen from the ashes, Louise." Next, Claire's "I guess burning all those candles for you paid off, my friend," tells me that I have ex-colleagues, now super-friends. Mona pours me another coffee and adds, "I really missed your laughter when you left; I can see that you haven't lost it. Good for you."

My mind is very alert and vibrant this morning as I remember so many faces, so many deep memories, all warm and soothing, of a time when I "lived" in this school. I can crack jokes, be witty and be wise with my mind; it simply needs a lot of rest to be able to function at peak capacity. No emotional roller coaster these days, but rather a smooth riding of the waves that are common to all of us whether we are challenged or merely alive. My Power lifts me, supports me, propels me to inspire others. I am spiritually fulfilled and my "jug" runneth over. I have a purpose in this world, a goal, a sense of what I still need to accomplish before I retire into the eternal life.

This morning, I experience a peaceful and moving excursion down memory lane. I am well.

As I wheel down the corridor, I dance in my head. I hear the high-heeled shoes of a former student, now "living" in this school.

My Dance

I have lived with chronic illness all of my life. Multiple sclerosis is a chronic illness that is familiar to me from a caregiver's perspective as well as from the position of one who actually has it. Neither of the roles has been easy for me, one has not been harder than the other. I think that whether one is a patient or a caregiver, there is an astonishing resemblance in the way in which we live our lives. Pain is pain, grieving is grieving, and reconstruction is reconstruction. The angle from which one comes is irrelevant, I believe. At the age of 36, my life was interrupted by multiple sclerosis. It is a time that is carved in my memory, a time when I felt the complex mystery of my own MS. Until then, my relationship with MS had been in the role of caregiver to my father who suffered with the disease for 27 years.

My diagnosis progressed in standard fashion from possible, to probable, to definite. The "probable" sentence was handed down to me around 11:00 at night. With a flashlight shining in my face, the neurologist awakened me in my hospital bed. There exists a blank space in my conscious memory of what precisely happened at that moment. Did I cry? Did I call someone on the telephone? Did I vomit? I suspect that if I did have a sensory memory, it would be of such horrific dimension that I could not handle it. I think of this coping mechanism as my fuse box, that simply shuts down, rather than catch on fire.

The next day, my family physician came on his regular rounds. With him, I was able to unfreeze somewhat, just enough to demand a second opinion. So began my series of jaunts to the MS clinic where I still maintain an active status. Ironically, this is the same clinic where my father was diagnosed, 36 years before me. A sense of eerieness came over me when I first wheeled around in the corridors wondering if my father had lain on a stretcher in this hall or that hall. With repeated visits to this same clinic, I have claimed my personal history with MS and not my father's story with the same disease.

With multiple sclerosis, the diagnosis is extremely tedious and is finalized by a process of elimination. To my good fortune, it took a brief six months, until the final "definite" diagnosis was pronounced. At first I always said, "It seems that I have MS." The use of "it seems" was the only way I could verbalize it at all. There did come a day, months later, when I summoned enough courage to say, "I have MS."

As with the first probable diagnosis, I have no vivid memory of the moments that followed my visit that day. I do remember wanting to see the MRI results; I needed to see my name in print on top of the report. Only then I would believe that I had multiple sclerosis. The shock wore off progressively. It seemed appropriate that in this particular month of January, nature had frozen outside my bedroom window. As I agonized through those first few months, I followed the natural path of all creation and rose from the ashes in the spring.

I emerged slowly from my petrified tomb of isolated fears. With the dance of the spring flowers, I too began to dance with rebirth; I joined the MS society because I realized that, "If you can't beat IT, join them who have IT."

I believe that *We are who we were.* In my own story, as well as in the stories of countless others that I have met or treated, chronic illness affects one's life but there still remains the basic thread of who we are. The illness, which often plays the role of the perfect excuse, is simply an added challenge. And so, just as I had always done, I prepared for battle.

The first order of business in the area of challenge was driving independently. I could not feel my feet. Dr. Bill could not give a prognosis on how long it would be until I could drive again. I had hired a young girl, Lorraine, to chauffeur me around. However, this elegant style did nothing for me. Soon, I could not live with this dependency any longer. After about six weeks, I had a hand-control installed in my car. Lorraine drove me to the hand-control supplier. On the way I said to her, "Did I ever tell you that I have my father's driver's license in my jewelry box at home? He gave it to me when I got my driver's license." For 27 years, Papa was driven to hospital examinations, visits with family, and on rare occasions a one-day ride. I needed to drive to reclaim my independence, the energy to sustain my mental and emotional health in the fight against this disease.

In one hour I accustomed myself to the new limb on my car; I was determined to be in control again. If this disease would take some things away from me, then I would change other things in order to accommodate those losses. But I would never give in to MS.

During a regular examination, as Dr. Bill pricked my feet with sharp needles, I responded, "Were you touching my foot at all?"

He answered, "Your MS is exacerbating again, Louise."

My MS? When did this become my MS? Painfully aware of the crucial need to own the disease if I were to tame and control it, I resigned myself. "Okay. It's my MS."

During the first years of my chronic illness, I had vowed to tame the illness, to own it, but never to *become* it nor to allow it to take over my entire life. It would mean a great deal of negotiation and I feared the undertaking. Someone introduced me to Bernie Siegel, the American "healer" who medically and emotionally treats people who are chronically or terminally ill. I voraciously read Siegel, this leading international authority on "living well." Soon, I began to think of myself as an exceptional patient – a term he uses to reflect his philosophy for ill persons (I believe that everyone has this capacity to be an exceptional person/patient, because it is the godlikeness in all of us.)

My dance with multiple sclerosis has been a ballroom dance, a polka, a fox trot, or a tango; with ease, stomping rhythm or sensuous flow. At times when I could not cope, when I isolated myself and froze, I sought professional help from therapists. I was floating around for the first few years, having lost my "feet on the ground" type of leverage. I had not landed yet.

The process could not be accelerated and believe me, I was not the most patient person. I was aware of not living the way I had in the past. I was not happy in my present and I was most terrified of my future. One of my identity problems was that I was not physically well, but not severely impaired; I sat on a fence between looking good and feeling quite awful. It was confusing at times for me. One therapist advised me to be flexible and to ride the waves of time. That worked well for a short time but it did not help matters that MS has the hallmark of unpredictability.

At the age of 36, I underwent a severe identity crisis. My career in teaching ended and I *marched* the Dance Macabre. Teaching had been my life, my vocation and a major source of fulfilment. I knew no other way of being. I wasn't a teacher anymore. Who was I now? My self-esteem was molded around situational factors, those concerned with "doing," rather than core factors, concerned with "being." *I was what I did.* Once MS interrupted the doing, I was nothing.

During this identity crisis, I developed my comedic self as a way of surviving my hospital incarcerations. I used laughter. When the nurse saw me come out of the bathroom with the measuring bowl for my urine on my head, she laughed and so did I. "Hey, can you get me another size-8 catheter, sweetie; how I long to be a size 8." With the humiliating interventions, I pranced around with laughter.

Dr. Bill reported in a serious tone, " Louise, this looks like the beginning of a paralysis on the left side: left face, left arm, left hand, left leg..."

"Hey, Doc, not the left brain I hope. I'm in the middle of a manuscript!"

During the sleepless nights, I strolled the halls. Usually it was when a nurse shut my door that I got up. The eerie shutting of the door that announces that someone has died was a loud speaker in my ears. My night walks took me to the smoke pit: "Hey, puffing away your misery! Ah! Let me get a whiff of that drug!"

In the television room friendships were born. "I respect you for staying here overnight; actually, it's the best way for you to grieve her right now; of course, you're angry, your wife is a beautiful 45-year-old woman, the woman of your life, and cancer is raping her, robbing her of that life. Yes, of course, we'll keep in touch, Dave, call me anytime."

Every time I went home again, I took with me the gifts of the people who glided into my life.

I believe that a hospital is not a place to be when you're sick. When I have to, when my condition becomes exacerbated, I do the required time and, as quickly as possible, go home to heal. I have grandiose ideas of how we could make hospitals into real healing places. Personal masseuses, large screen television sets, Internet, sound systems, jacuzzis, Abbott and Costello video library, hors d'oeuvres and fine wine, private love-making rooms, orderlies in tuxedos, and the list goes on.

I live painstakingly through my hospital visits with music, meditation, and a massive dose of Bernie Siegel at my bedside. The cleaning lady's mop hitting on my bed, the nurse delivering medications every few hours, the telephone ringing for my roomy, the visitors chattering, the library person, the senile woman chatting at my bedside – all of these are noise. The eerieness of the night with its deafening silence, the announcement of death with the closing of the patient's door, the lament of the suffering, the pacing of loved ones – all of these are unsettling. Always, it is the dancing party when I go home, relieved to be back in my healing place. Our home is adapted as we need it, with privacy, flowers, music, warm bubble baths, and of course, my healing canine.

During the course of my chronic illness, I have suffered from retention of urine; this means that I need to catheterize in order to avoid dangerous infection. This is, by far, the most humiliating exercise I have had to experience. First I needed lessons on how to do the deed appropriately; that in itself was no picnic. Then, my husband needed to be trained since, at times, my hands cannot function well enough to perform the task. My sexuality suffers from these episodes, reminding me of all that I take for granted.

Sometimes, we the challenged are intolerable people, angry and raging or depressed and teary. We are violated over and over again by the disease with which we struggle. Our families need to know that it takes time for us to become friendly and approachable once more and even longer to become our own best friends.

Somehow I manage to keep the black holes in my life from scarring my professional life. To most people, I am a symbol of sunshine and optimism. I do fear my depression a great deal, even though I perform well in public. As I look back, I recognize that there were times when my survival hung by a thread. The emotional bleakness that I experienced reached suicidal proportions in those first few years.

At root, I know today, I am not a depressive individual but an intense one. This intensity can extend itself in any direction and my MS is synonymous to depression. I have learned to dance with both. I have persisted in delving into self-discovery and have attempted to always benefit from the loving support of those who have multiple sclerosis. When I violate the limit of how much intensity I can handle, I gently swing back toward a balanced center.

I suffer from organic depression, which is very symptomatic of MS. It was a tug of war for me to accept medication until this state of depression had passed. Somehow, I had old tapes playing in my head that claimed that taking medication for depression is a sign of weakness. The journey to this realization that depression is an illness and not something I can do much about, followed by the acceptance of it, has been tedious. It warms my heart to know that there are physicians, psychiatrists and other caregivers who take the time to attend to their patients by explaining the difference between organic, situational, and manic depression.

A major concern for me was the possibility that my depression would affect my professional life. I perform a lot and act "as if," which is natural for me. When I become aware of my depression, the stage lights go on; when I leave my nest-like home the performance begins. This strategy is of therapeutic value because the time spent away is refreshing for me. One of the best treatments for depression is to keep going as if the inner world is sunshiny.

There is value and assistance to be had in talking about one's depression to someone during the course of chronic illness. It appears that once something is named and owned, it loses some of its power. Secrets are powerful and they weigh us down. Connecting with another person, for me, has been an experience of dividing the pain, of allowing a crack in the wall of my isolation. I suspect that a listener who has some experience with the illness and with depression is better equipped for compassionate empathy.

The physical challenge of MS as it relates to vision has forced me to choreograph new dances with my eyes. Usually I sense a strange sensation, sometimes burning, sometimes even pain. I usually wait a few hours until Dr. Bill is available to check my eyes. Once, as he examined my eyes as part of a general physical examination, he found optic neuritis. Two hours later, I was hospitalized for a steroid treatment.

This particular treatment is Solu-Medrol administered by IV. It makes me crazy. I hear bells and the telephone ringing; usually I get very depressed and excessively bloated. But I don't ever gamble with my eyes. Both my husband, who happens to be legally blind, and I know the great need we have for one good pair of eyes between us.

When my vision worsens, I often become protective of my feeling world. I crack jokes incessantly as a means of deflecting the harsh reality. Terror and rage begin a two-step dance. These emotions can be of overwhelming proportions. Sometimes my sense of humor, often parading as sarcasm, joins in the dance.

Whether for a change in my eyes or for a change in any other physical manifestation of my MS, the waiting game is always a challenge. Waiting kills me since I am structured and impatient.

One of the most difficult factors with my MS is its unpredictability. In the middle of meetings, when we have plans to go somewhere, in the heart of a telephone conversation or just about at any given moment, I can notice a warning that something is amiss. Sometimes it's a tingle, a numbness, a burning, a weakness. Since I do not want to become paranoid with this disease, *who* has become a lifelong companion, I tend to ignore the first signs or symptoms until they are prolonged. Often, my husband assists me in monitoring these signals and in doing so, we do not neglect the warnings that persist.

The people close to me are by this time educated and know that I am consistently chameleon-like as far as my commitments go. Still, I accept invitations as though I did not have a chronic illness because I refuse to live under its domination. My vision of tomorrow is one with no limitations; if and when they arise, I accommodate them accordingly. I have met too many persons who allow chronic illness to take over their lives. They become the disease. My stubbornness and tenacity forbid my surrendering my life to MS. So my husband and I plan many trips, most of which we take. We plan for success not for failure.

At the beginning of my challenge with chronic illness, I experienced things differently than I do today, eight years later. Everything happened above the shoulders. That is, I had a cognitive, medical, and robotic type of approach and coping mechanism. I ordered the latest medical research from England but it did nothing for my emotional survival and, to some extent, not much for my spiritual well-being. I spoke to various exceptional persons to find out their secret for quality of life. Siegel became my main source of inspiration on how to live *with* an illness, as opposed to how to live *as* an illness. Now I consider myself an exceptional patient on most days.

I have the exacerbation/remission form of multiple sclerosis. Dr. Bill is always supportive in my recoveries. As I reclaim my strength after each attack, he is beside me on the upward climb. With repetition, we learn the most we can from each incident. I find it amazing how the months following a relapse are a gradual crawl back to where I was before. It is painful to realize that I lose a little each time, a little that I never get back. My ultimate goal is to recycle myself to the state I was in before an attack, but often it does not work that way. I remain positive and diligent nevertheless.

There is little time to think or worry during the first few weeks following an exacerbation. Those days fly by: the hospitalization, the influx of well-wishers, the medication treatment. Then, at a slower pace, the crawling begins: the adjustment and the reprogramming.

Whether we want to or not, we become pros and make a conscious effort to transform our home into a healing place following each attack. We have an intercom system in the house so that I feel safe; I tend to become terrorized by everything when MS strikes. Because visuals are important to me, we try to keep the house well decorated with flowers; out come my special healing comforter for television watching and whichever stuffed toy I need for protection.

My dog, Bartholomew-Moisha is a healing presence. Each time I feel sluggish, he follows me around the house like a caretaker. He licks my hand if I cry and snuggles next to me in bed. His unconditional love means a lot to me. There are times I say things to him that I would not say to any other living soul. One time, he developed a painful eye infection when I had optic neuritis; I thought he had a sympathetic disease.

I am determined not to become an angry woman raging at her losses. I must work diligently and consistently. I look at what I have, I am grateful for what I am left with after each attack. I make lemonade out of the lemons. I gambol through the loss of mobility, bladder control, bowel function, sight, short-term memory, and hair. More importantly, I prance with the "what is left" list: a sound intellect, some mobility, dexterity to type, hair regrowth, catheters that fit properly, natural herbs for the bowel, corrective lenses, Post-it notes to help me remember.

It would be easy to fall into the trap of letting my whole world revolve around MS and to become an MS person. I am not. I am a woman who happens to have MS. However, it is with love that I have and maintain an active status with the MS Society. Some of the issues concerning MS are frightening to me. In my work with the society, it is not always easy or possible to disassociate my name from the list of those in chronic progressive states. The individuality factor saves me, since everyone can experience his or her own course differently with the Mighty Strange disease.

When I give a seminar for the MS society, as a guest speaker, I become both elated at being able to contribute and at the same time emotional from witnessing the effects of this chronic illness on people. For me there is a sense of responsibility in speaking for the cause of my illness. I speak in the name of those who are afflicted and cannot speak, either because MS has robbed them of their voice or because they are overwhelmed by their emotional challenge.

It has happened that I have been caught off guard seeing my name printed in a newspaper under the heading of "MS." As if I wake up at moments and think, "When did all this happen?" Soon enough, reality sets in and I begin to remember the first time my limbs were numb, the first time the neurologist pricked my feet, the first time my vision blurred, and the first time I spoke the words, "I have multiple sclerosis..."

When any member of my family is present at an MS function where I speak, the talk takes on a special flavor. As with many families, my family has an unspoken rule about not disclosing too much around illness; we are all great dancers. I am certain that our cotillion was born with the destruction of our father's health and identity, with the colossal changes that the whole family unit underwent, and with identifying ourselves as a family with MS. We protect each other. Although we feel deeply for one another, we can remain superficial at times; the distance is a defense mechanism against pain, an attitude that proclaims, "keep a stiff upper lip." I have come to understand that my family, like so many others, need time to learn the choreography of the dance: their suffering, their compassion, and their love.

Each individual member lives the illness differently. What care giving means to one sibling can be different than what it means for another sibling; one can smother while the other can become disengaged. It is an intricate pattern of temperaments, from the easy-going to the stressed out, each person's unique signature personalizing what is happening to him. Some conflict can arise in this area and we need to make constant attempts to accept this facet of family interactions. How does it feel for the challenged one to be singled out? How does it feel for the care-giving sibling to see the ill one? Often, I have shied away from opening up to members of my family, because it hurts me twice as much; I hurt for me and I hurt for them.

For My Brothers and My Sisters...

I Cannot Tell You

If I cannot tell you of my pain
it is because
Then, I hurt twice upon utterance
As I see my pain reflected in your face,
I feel like the creator
Of the pain you feel through me.

When I reach such despair
To tell you is to remain alive.

And in the aftermath of our reciprocal pain
Comes a healing and a serenity.

My husband, my primary caregiver, and I ballroom dance; we are often interrupted by multiple sclerosis, who stomps in uninvited and unannounced. "For better or for worse, in sickness or in health...Are you sure, Mel? Yes. Are you sure, Louise? Yes." The memory of my husband's face when we spoke those words to each other is my constant beacon of admiration for him.

I fought him before our wedding: "I could be in a wheelchair permanently. You might have to wipe my bum when my hands shake. I may lose my sight also." He never budged. He has never, in these our first ten years together, budged.

I made a point of educating him about what could happen in the course of this chronic illness. It *did* take effort on both our parts for him to understand where I was coming from: "Let me decide which nightgown I want to wear today or if I want to take such a drug." I spoke of my power, my choices, my need to keep my independence. Where does care giving become too much like smothering? What happens between the dance partners when one overprotects the other?

Sometimes he jumps in too quickly at the onset of symptoms; this is because he is not experiencing the physiological challenge. "It's not time to call Dr. Bill yet, the burning in my arm is just a symptom right now." I usually wait before I notify my physician since it has been my experience that many symptoms persist and nothing serious comes of them. For the caregiver, who has vivid images of the potential of the disease, each symptom is more frightening. "Why are you so stubborn, Louise? It's getting late, we have to go and put you to bed." We need to practice continually on the ballroom floor, to change the music once in a while, to dress up for the evening ball.

I have known many couples who, unfortunately, have not made it through the challenge of dancing with chronic illness. For most couples whose relationship is based on activities and a life-style with an "abled" partner, chronic debilitating illness upsets the dynamics. Once the husband or the wife becomes challenged, all the rules change. I consider myself extremely fortunate to have a husband who has not known me other than as the heel kicker with MS.

At the time of my diagnosis, my son was eight years old. He grieved the loss of my health. A few months into the illness, I walked in on him one day. He stood in front of the couch in the living room, his face red with rage, his whole body engaged in beating the couch with my canes. It was as though all of his pain, his helplessness, his fear, his rage possessed him for those few moments. The canes were his catalyst as he beat the couch violently. "It's okay, Adam, to be angry...I am too. Sometimes I just cry instead of getting really mad like this." He remained silent, ceased the beating, and left the room. In my mind, my heart, and my body, I hurt. "What is this vile disease doing to my son? Oh, God, he's hurting so much. Shit! I just wet myself again!"

He tried to take care of me by not going out to play with his friends. Knowing full well that this was not a healthy way for a child to spend his free time, I always encouraged him to live his childhood, to play and have a ball. One afternoon, he snuck up on me; I was crying.

"Come on, Mommy, let's play cards."

"Hey, didn't Marty want you to ride your bicycle with him? Well, out you go. Adam, I'm still the mommy and you're still the little boy... you go out and play and I'll take care of myself."

The fact that I had to take care of my father when I was a child helped me to understand that I could and I would provide my son with a normal childhood. Even though at times it has been frightening for him and for me, I have told him the truth about my condition and what is happening with my body from time to time. It is a relief to observe the healthy attitude he has developed toward the challenged population. I feel such colossal pride when I observe him giving a seminar in his law class about "The rights and the dignity of the challenged." With hard work and courage, we step to the music.

The greatest sadness of all: millions of challenged persons must "dance with chronic illness" along with me. My story is not unusual. One day we cope well and have a good quality of life; the next day we succumb to the emotional challenge and cry all day; the day after that we curse the Power that may be for afflicting us with chronic illness. There is nothing fair about chronic illness. It just is.

I try not to hit my head against the wall or to use my energy in areas where there is nothing to be gained. The people that share my life also share my strife from their perspective as best they can. When I run away from them because it hurts too much, they usually come to fetch me. In most things, I attempt to keep my power of choice and my dignity of life. There is so much to be changed out there, in the "un-challenged world," and I truly believe that it has to come from me, from us, the challenged.

Many of us are hard on ourselves; we forget to take care of ourselves or we think we are not worth the effort since we are less-abled. I attempt not to fall into that trap, although let me assure you, it is difficult. Whether it's wearing beautiful lingerie, eating fine foods, vacationing, or doing any other "self-care" activity that I can, all assist me in maintaining a positive outlook and a confident definition of my true self. Never do I want pity, but empathy and compassion are acceptable. I trust in my power to go through whatever the dance with chronic illness entails and when I need to rest, I trust in myself to do just that. I am not only who I was before MS. I am more than I have ever been.

TWO

Grieving

The Old Dance

The Flower

I am buried under deep snow.
I am heavy, numb, yet alive.
Bitterly broken
I rage, I despair.

Gifted with winter.
Frozen in glacial grief.
Stilled in the hope of my soul.
I will rise again.

Grieving, a growth process, is necessary if we are to achieve quality living in spite of chronic illness. Grieving is a prerequisite to mental health. In effect, we surrender the old life and make way for the new life. Typically, grieving is characterized by powerful emotions such as shock, denial, anger, rage, resentment, fear, sadness and guilt. We need to remember that grieving is a passage: the way out of the old, a conduit to the new, in essence, a birth canal. The challenge borne of the grieving process may reside in its repetitive character, brought on by triggers or by aggravated, illness-related conditions.

As we observe and attend to persons who suffer from chronic illness, and who are grieving as a result, we often witness their extremely bleak turmoil; grieving can be all-consuming. Certain factors come into play, such as the degree of loss and level of mental and emotional resilience of the afflicted person. For those who are grieving, the process engulfs their life; there is no end in sight, no hope. The irony is that the more they can experience the losses, and their emotional reactions and responses to these losses, the greater their chances are of coming out on the other side, into a new life. Caregivers should always encourage verbalization and the communication of the grieving process from those who are submerged in it. We need not give in to our own fears, which is a natural tendency; the idea is to allow the grieving person to do their task completely and effectively and to attend to them effectively.

For many of us, the concept of grief was defined within the confines of death: natural, physical death. We have come to realize that grief is the natural outcome of any and all loss. Daily we come into contact with loss; at intervals, we lose bigger pieces of what used to be. A son will leave home for university, a co-worker will transfer, our hair will begin to grey, our pet cat will pass on, we will divorce our partner or our body will begin to show signs of aging. The losses cause the grieving.

Whatever we lose needs to be owned by our feeling dimension, let go of, and then replaced. This void-like experience is one that we often observe or live through when grieving begins. It is as though part of being human is longing to fill the voids in our lives. Thus, when an empty space is all that remains of something that used to be, like a relationship or a physical characteristic or some material possession, we hurt until that void becomes filled with something or someone else. Therein lies the danger of going through the grieving process too quickly, compulsively filling this void as hastily as possible. We, as human beings, fear pain and so we fear grieving.

Too often, we do not fully appreciate what we have until we lose it. When the grieving begins, the pain is a direct product of coming to the realization of what we had, and the possible guilt surrounding our nonchalance over what we had.

Elisabeth Kübler-Ross, the mother of modern study of the grieving process, wrote *On Death and Dying*. She described grief as a natural process and "normalized" it for many of us who were socialized not to talk about it. The stages of grief, which she defined, describe extremely well what happens to us when we become chronically ill.

The caregiver to the chronically challenged person experiences their own grieving process. Even though the losses may be indirect or different than those lived by the patient, the losses are of the same magnitude. It is possible for a partner of an ill person to grieve even more intensely than the partner directly afflicted. One determining factor is the capacity for enduring and rising above emotional pain, and the willingness to get on with life. The more effectively one grieves, the more one is actually getting on with the business of living. We cannot arrive in Paris until we leave home behind us; we cannot begin to live again, be it very differently than before, until we have abandoned our former life.

We yearn for our former energy so that we can climb the few stairs to our bedroom without stopping and sitting on the steps. We cry over the loss of friends who fear their own fragility. We rage when we need to insert the painful catheter that will bring our mechanical voiding. We are horrified at the dozens of pill bottles in our cabinet. We long to walk again, without a cane, without help from someone supporting us. We do not remember the last time we enjoyed sex. We doubt that we possess any worth at all.

However, we are who we were in that our natural temperament is not altered by chronic illness, although the *way* in which we live, the way in which we relate to ourselves and to others may, of necessity, change. The paraplegic who used to run must mourn his inability to run the marathon before he opens himself to a new way of fulfilling his need for activity. If he mourns the marathon while he envisions his healthy body running with the wind, then his grief seems insurmountable; only when he surrenders to the knowledge that he will not run again is he ready to be something different.

What follows are the stages of grieving as I perceive them and have experienced them.

Stages of Grieving

1. I can't believe IT...
   I am frozen in shock — SHOCK

2. I won't believe IT...
   I am numbed with sadness — DEPRESSION

3. I am ready to look at IT...
   I am resentful and angry — ANGER

4. I am moving towards IT...
   I am frightened — FEAR

5. I dance with IT...
   I am recycled — ACCEPTANCE

He's Out of It

from Bob's wife's diary

I am so concerned about Bob; it's like he's on another planet. Ever since we received the diagnosis, he talks incessantly about chronic fatigue. And because he has no energy, all he does is sleep and read all this stuff about his illness; medical updates, medication trials, even quack cures. When I ask him how he feels about the whole thing, after a brief, "Fine," he mumbles a bit about what he's been reading.

Everything has happened so quickly with him, I wonder if he realizes what this disease means to all of us in this family? A lot of our friends keep dropping in on him and he does the same type of major avoidance with them.

He has not even cried or been depressed the way I expected he would be. I was so angry yesterday, and I let it all out, threw around a few pots and pans and slammed the door to the bedroom. After a good cry I felt I had at least let some of the strangling feeling in my throat out. As I did that, Bob seemed not even connected to what I was going through. His only comment: "That won't get you anywhere."

What Marcia is reporting is the first stage of grieving. This initial phase is *shock*.

In this stage, a person experiences a natural anesthetic; perhaps nature cares for us in this way. People in this stage cannot allow themselves to believe that they are afflicted. "This can't be happening to me." The fact that illness has hit so close to home is unbelievable; many do not allow themselves to deal with it and especially not to feel. At this point, denial predominates; we go on with our lives, sometimes as if nothing has occurred.

Bob's ongoing frenzy, which Marcia reports, typifies the *shock* stage. Many of us search out the libraries and medical institutions for every possible word ever written about the disease. We make lists and decisions about our adaptation, unfortunately way too soon. Panic strikes. The mind seeks out rapid solutions to the problem. Being in this cognitive mode reduces the feeling self; no emotional pain is acknowledged. Patients recite how they will conquer this problem, and seemingly have all the answers. The blind expect to see again, the HIV positive will beat the odds, and the paralyzed will walk again.

At this time, we keep ourselves occupied with the physical dimension: medical tests, medical treatments and forms to fill. The business at hand clutters our lives with "to do" items; we freeze in time. Both psychologically and physically, the person affected may have a decreased ability to respond to others in his usual manner. A lot of energy may be spent on trying to contain the panic which has struck.

The shock stage is similar to posttraumatic shock syndrome. We need to respect this part of the process as being therapeutical. A brief interval of time precedes recognition of the reality, the acknowledgement of the situation. No one prepares for chronic illness. The astonishment at the possibility of having a chronic illness sets off this anesthetic mode, protecting us from feeling a reality that would be otherwise unlivable.

Usually in a couple system, the partner in the care-giving role will observe his or her mate in the shock stage as Marcia did with Bob. Marcia's own shock time might occur later when she begins to realize the magnitude of the events that are taking place. She is being strong for Bob, while *shock* cushions him.

Down and Out
from Sarah's diary

I am too depressed to cry. My energy is zapped. I live in a black hole. An albatross hangs around my neck, an albatross named lupus. I find refuge in my bed. I pull the covers over my head and sleep for hours on end. I am alone. There are people around, but no one is actually in this black hole with me. Nothing excites me. The things that used to raise my spirits, like David talking about a trip to Europe, just don't do it anymore. Yesterday, he mentioned that maybe a cruise would lift my spirits. I said "whatever." Every morning, I drag myself out of bed and realize that the black hole is still there; no sunshine can reach me. I feel dead.

Actually, being dead would probably be a relief. My illness has taken over my entire life; I can't go to work, I am a nobody. I feel like I am a crippled woman with a sick heavy mind and a frozen heart. I thought that by now, four months after my diagnosis, I would get over the sadness. At the beginning, the diagnosis didn't really bother me as much as it does now; I don't understand. Who cares anyway. I have not got the mental energy to figure this out.

•

Sarah's comments reflect the *depression* stage. It takes over after some initial shock and denial has worn off, usually a few months after the onset of chronic illness or its diagnosis. By this time, the well-wishers have ceased to visit, the flowers have all died, and the "get-well" cards have stopped arriving. Of course, people in our lives have come to terms with the helplessness that they experience in trying to change what has happened to us.

Some forms of depression are organic and a direct result of neurological and other physiological conditions; a competent physician can shed some light on the depression. If the state manifests as a chemical reaction to the illness, then proper medication can be administered to offset it. When we are dealing with situational depression brought on by the circumstances due to this new challenge, some form of therapy is called for. A competent therapist would treat the patient with various behavioral techniques, such as avoiding isolation, getting lots of fresh air, or journaling.

The depression stage forces the person challenged with chronic illness to consider the possibility of her illness, the actuality of it. Usually the smallest indication of being able to believe it brings, at the same time, a refusal to believe. In order to maintain this level of non-belief, one isolates; other people in his or her life may support the truth and the patient refuses or cannot handle this truth. With depression comes isolation. Isolated people tend to become unpleasant to be with. Thus, well-wishers or regular visitors cease to become involved with the challenged person.

Sarah mentions death as almost desirable at this time, however, she does not wish to die. Usually in depression, a person uses this reference only to communicate the felt insurmountability of this black hole. The person expresses their sorrow as a means to get out of the pit of despair. Death would be a relief, however, for depressed persons. It is the next stage, the anger stage that will summon the energy to actually attempt to die. During the depression stage, an attendant or family member should not overreact to the challenged person's reference to death, but simply respond to it by acknowledging how brutal the *depression* feels.

I Could Kill
from Leah's diary

Last night, I allowed my husband to coerce me into going to what would have been my 25th anniversary banquet as a teacher. I almost threw cake into a few faces that kept saying how good I look. I feel like shit...like shit...What am I supposed to do, look like hell so that they will attest to this f—ing condition?

I gave the best 18 years of my life to that job and what do I have to show for it, shit. No trophy, not even any verbal recognition of what I was for those students. I hate them all for ignoring me this way. When they took a photograph of the "gang" no one even thought of including me in it. They can all rot in hell!

When we got home, I let my husband have it! I told him in no uncertain terms to stay the hell out of my life. From now on, I will be a hermit if I wish. He has no idea of what this is like. I am a living corpse. I have been raped by this MS, violated to the very core. I honestly believe that if I had a loaded gun, right now, I would blow my head off.

Leah rages in pain. *Anger* is the next stage of the challenge of grieving . She experienced her rage when an event triggered the sorrow buried in her subconscious for some time. Events such as an anniversary, a phone call, an article in a newspaper or meeting someone can trigger anger and rage. Rage is a more serious degree of anger, one that is usually played out in behavior, such as shouting, throwing objects, or even violent acts.

Anger, an emotional reaction to a primary emotion, acts as a defense against pain or fear; through anger, we cope with that fear. Anger is neither a positive nor a negative emotion. It's just an emotion. It can range from mild irritation to full blown rage as in suicide. Unfortunately, anger can mask itself as depression, sarcasm or humor. Repressed anger can create physiological conditions such as heart disease. Anger adds to the chronically ill person's already serious potential for isolation.

Anger stems from a sense of loss of control and chronic illness is all about loss of control. It may come in waves or may stay for longer periods of time. The high intensity of the anger from a chronically challenged person is a response to the "no-win" situation.

Anger will be vented once the depression lifts. At this stage, the person will search out a target to blame or to rage at. This can be very healthy and more than that, quite necessary to achieve effective grieving. Things to consider are effective anger processing techniques, those which do not harm anyone, neither the patient nor the people in their lives. If the anger reaches raging proportions, it can be monitored to assure that it is healthily and effectively processed.

If the challenged person begins to turn the rage inward, this can result in suicide – the ultimate in self-destruction. When a challenged person represses and denies their anger, they can become severely depressed or lethargic. We will do well to seek professional help and assistance in order to live through the anger and rage in an appropriate way. We want to avoid an uncontrolled, unmonitored letting go of the raging anger.

Choosing an anger coach is wise, in order to avoid mismanagement of anger symptoms. Someone who knows the situation, who has proven in the past to have effective anger management skills would be preferable. Professional help is most often recommended, especially if one feels stuck in the anger. Of course, we must give careful consideration when choosing help. Inappropriate expressions of anger must be avoided.

If the challenged person attacks their family, friends, or the medical staff, either physically, verbally or emotionally, it is inappropriate. Throwing things at people, hitting them, yelling obscenities at them or giving them the silent treatment, are all negative management techniques. If a challenged person harms themself by neglecting their condition or by not taking proper medication or taxing their body too much, they participate in negative anger management. By not owning up to the primary feelings such as sadness and fear that are underneath the anger they prolong the suffering. Therefore, effective investigation of the longevity of the anger is necessary. Here, the anger coach listens and teaches proper anger management skills.

How then can anger be managed effectively and healthily so as to provide healing for the challenged person? It is necessary to verbalize, either by speaking, or by writing and reading out loud, using raging words if necessary. Drawing a picture or finding one that expresses what we feel can be helpful. In the same fashion, we can draw a picture of our target and let the picture have the anger; we should never draw a picture of a person as a target for the anger. Engaging the body in venting the anger is usually comforting. Pound a pillow or other safe surface. Angry letters can serve to vent one's anger; we can tear them up afterward, or process their contents with someone.

It may sometimes be necessary for the challenged person to avoid hooking into others' anger; we become trapped into this, whether a person is challenged by chronic illness or not. Since networking with others who are also challenged is a good activity for the challenged person, there is more chance of getting caught up in another's battle. As a challenged person, we cannot afford to fight anyone else's battle. Time should be set aside to vent our anger; this will help us avoid being constantly in the anger mode. Anger energizes us emotionally. Many opportunities will surface that will allow us to channel or refocus this energy in a positive way, such as the rights of the physically challenged. Anger will be part of our grieving and so why not use its energy to maintain dignity and quality of living.

Anger triggers are external events or forces which cause or "trigger" a release or expression of anger. If the family or other support system seems to abandon the challenged person, this will trigger anger in the person afflicted. Even old resentments and unfinished business with others will surface at this time. Some anger triggers might be:

- the anniversary of the last "worked day"
- a wedding anniversary
- the anniversary of a divorce
- the anniversary of a diagnosis
- comparing one's self to others who are not so incapacitated

- an incident of financial stress
- an awareness of loss of family or social role
- a scene from a television show
- a song playing on the radio
- receiving a phone call
- an article in the newspaper
- a perceived violation of boundaries by a caregiver
- a lack of compassion from the "well" society.

Anger triggers in essence are common incidences; however, when they are experienced and perceived in the context of chronic illness, they may easily set off anger for the challenged individual.

Once a challenged person identifies the triggering factor connected to the anger, they at least become aware of the source. Next comes the more difficult part, taking responsibility for their anger and its effective management. Chronic illness does not give them a license to become a raging aggressor.

As in the case of all individuals, *I am responsible for my anger*, I am accountable for my anger. Just as we struggle to maintain power over our choice, especially when stricken with chronic illness, we are accountable for our anger and its effective management.

The attendant or the caregiver has a responsibility to be with us, the challenged person, as we process the anger but *they are not responsible to fix it, to change it or to suppress it.* One is responsible for his or her own self-care through this processing.

Although anger is more common in the lives of challenged persons than in the lives of "well" persons, the effective management of anger is exactly the same in both groups. Most importantly, *anger* is a healthy response to pain and to fear; it is an energy that a person can capitalize on and is a necessary part of grieving chronic illness.

I'm So Afraid

from Sarah's diary

I never have been so afraid of everything. It's been over one year now since the day of my diagnosis. Last Christmas, I was so depressed, I didn't go to my mom's for dinner; then, I wound up angry at my family because they did not understand. These days I am not angry or depressed, I am just frightened. I feel like a little fragile child, up for grabs.

Each time a symptom flares up, I start shaking inside, knowing full well what the potential is. Will I wake up with a pancreatitis attack? Will I be wriggling with the pain in my swollen knuckles? What if I become addicted to my pain medication? I fear that my husband will have an affair with someone else, because I'm never interested in sex and he always works late. I want him to hold me because I am so afraid. The road ahead is frightening...what if I stop breathing entirely during a bout of pleurisy? Ever since I saw that television star in a wheelchair, I have been so afraid of my own end.

There is so much unknown for me, and this disease is so strong when it takes over my body. The fact that I can't fight off a common cold tells me just how fragile I am. I get scared when someone rings the doorbell, when the phone rings, when my son yells down from his room, when I think I have upset my husband. I have never been so frightened of living.

What Sarah describes is a healthy part of grieving: *fear.* The challenged person has gained a considerable amount of awareness, more knowledge about the disease, has isolated and lived with anger, only to find a life strewn with fear. There is a definite tendency to experience ourselves as totally vulnerable and in need of protection from others. Challenged persons report needing their blankets around them, a sort of protective defense against the world. Understanding the possible progression of one's disease, whether by reading about it, by experiencing it, or, as in Sarah's case, by seeing someone on television who has it, can in fact generate tremendous fear that "this is happening to me too."

No doubt the shock stage is less threatening. Even the anger stage with its possibility of energy release is less intense. The fear stage happens when we get in touch with the harsh reality that we have fallen prey to a chronic illness. We fear dying painfully; every person with a chronic illness thinks about death in a way different from able-bodied persons. Financial insecurity creates fear of how we, as well as our family, will survive. Many marriages break down; inevitably, the fear of being cheated on enters our thoughts. Abandonment sits way at the top of the list of fears.

If a challenged person can express the fear, it diminishes somewhat. Expressing fear can be done successfully by dialoguing, writing, or imaging. No greater fear exists than facing fear on our own. Also, we can remember the slogan: "FEAR: False Evidence Appearing Real."

This stage is in effect one that is absolutely healthy and necessary in the grieving cycle. This does not make things any easier for the suffering person stuck in the fear. For the person experiencing the fear, a key antidote rests in validation by caregivers or others. The reality and rational expression of what is actually going on is best done through cognitive processing; caregivers will do well to attempt to reason with the challenged person. It does not mean that the challenged person cannot or should not experience fear, it simply means that the experience of the *fear* will subside more quickly if the person engages their logical mind in the process.

I Live Fully, My Disease Lives with Me
from Leah's diary

As I scooted along in the mall yesterday, I caught a glimpse of myself in a window; "you've come a long way baby." So I'm riding around instead of walking...kind of neat I think. My life is different than it was five years ago. Different, but just as good. The roller coaster ride has been quite an experience. In the war I live with my disease, I lose a few battles, but I will not lose the war. I still have bad moments, bad days; sometimes on the pity-pot or raging for a few moments. But on the whole, I have tamed this beast of a disease. I love myself again, respect myself, prize myself and my integrity above all else.

My life is filled with activity, different sorts of readings and projects that I would not have done prior. I have discovered talents that I never knew I had. More than that, I have discovered an inner life that I never took time to tap into before. I do not live with my disease, I live and IT lives with me.

Leah has arrived at the summit of her grieving cycle: *acceptance*. In contrast with the "peaceful waters, everything is perfect " type of imagery that the term conjures up, acceptance is born of the actual tempestuous sea where one has to sail to get to the calm waters. It is a place one comes to after a long climb through numbed feelings, tears and fears.

A sense of peace accompanies this final stage where there seems to be an ability to "just go on with living" minus the losses. Persons display creativity at this stage, innovative ways of coping and living with a healthy degree of contentment. Acceptance with resignation is hopelessness; *acceptance* with a sense of purpose in life is what we seek. *We dance with the illness.*

It is common for a challenged person to experience the various stages of grieving more than once. For example, any remission in the illness will produce denial and a new false sense of truth. Of course, when the illness takes its course once again, the person goes back to step one: shock. In most cases, the second, third or subsequent times into depression, for example, will not be as lengthy nor as profoundly draining as the initial experience of depression. Especially when a person has the knowledge that the painful stage has ended before, there is hope that it will end again.

THREE

The Physical Challenge

Our Bodies in the Dance

The Treatment

Drip...drip...drip...

To my invader, welcome, I have unlatched the door.
I abhor your violation and your rape
yet
I invite your magic potion.

As each of your drops burn their way in my veins
Your fire rampages through my body.
The slow rhythm of your falling temperament
Its macabre drum dance of wildfire.

Yet

You have proven yourself able to outwit my disease
Stop it in its tracks, even if only for brief intervals.
You render me more cautious since I have come to know you,
Your potential to harm, your pain, your healing.

You are cordially invited
To dwell within the cavities of my temple
and
At every moment lived in ecstasy of G-d's creation
When my alive eyes sing praise
I will speak well of you.

Medications

The poem that introduces this chapter on "physical challenge" is intended to give a glimpse into the effects of certain medications used during the course of a chronic illness. Indeed, a drug treatment is an invasion of one's body. The particular drug spoken of here is a potent steroid administered intravenously for five consecutive days.

Now for the bad news. While using this drug, the patient usually requires hospitalization because of the possible complications. The drip must be perfectly regulated as it enters the patient's vein, or the patient will suffer excruciating burning in the hand and arm. Pain and treatment become synonymous. After the first few days of the treatment, the entry spot can get severely swollen and bruised, therefore the needle needs to be moved into another part of the patient's limb. Still this is not the worst news.

The most challenging part of this treatment is its emotional and psychological impact on the patient. The drug, like narcotics and other corticosteroids, plays havoc on the mood center and can even alter the personality of the patient. It may cause a false sense of well-being, whereby the patient "floats" around only to severely crash once the treatment is over. Some side effects include the hearing of bells, buzzing in the ears, extensive hyperactivity (such as wanting to wash walls all night long), severe insomnia, anxiety and acute depression, to mention only a few.

For people living with chronic illness, medications are simply a fact of life. And while drug interventions come with unwanted side effects, what are the options? For an MS patient, the decision to wait it out or to refuse Solu-Medrol, for example, may mean partial or complete loss of sight. For those dancing with other chronic illnesses, the names of the drugs, the side effects, and the consequences of refusing the intervention may all be different but the issues surrounding acceptance and refusal of drug interventions are the same. The choice to be made, the alternative of refusing such drug interventions, demands serious consideration from the person affected. Some physicians, if we are lucky, will consult with us and give us the ultimate power to decide yes or no.

If the patient is to claim their power of choice and is capable of making a conscious and informed decision, then it would be the ideal situation for them to do so. However, in too many cases, the physicians make the decisions, with little consideration for the point of view of the patient, or simply because they do not have the time or the energy to educate the patient prior to the need to make such a decision. Once again, the need for a person to become familiar with their chronic illness, the possible treatments and what each entails remains the responsibility of the person with the chronic illness. If the physician observes this attitude in the patient, then the chances are greater that the physician will allow the patient to make the final decision.

Illness is powerful. Therefore, any amount of power that can be taken back by a patient, any choice that can be made by the patient, contributes to the sense of taking the lead.

At the same time, we must recognize the potential bind the whole dynamic places the patient in. We risk being labeled difficult if we demand our power. In most instances, the premise is that the doctor is the expert. However, if we first validate that expertise, we can inquire from the physician with a clear and direct understanding that we genuinely strive to become more medication literate. Building a patient/doctor relationship demands courage and time. By communicating to our doctor the emotional impact of the physiological problem, we can create an atmosphere of partnership wherein we take on our power and make educated choices about medication. We aim to work *with* our doctor, in a combined effort, for our wellness.

Because many treatments involve a high dose of drug to be ingested, the aftermath – the withdrawal – is part of the challenge for the person. When you consider the fact that certain treatments can last for weeks, even months, it is understandable that one's body can become "addicted" to this drug. Now comes the withdrawal and all of the adjustments that this entails. If the drug has had a positive effect on the person, for example prednisone which often gives a "high" to the person taking it, then one has to adjust to not having this stimulant any longer. If the drug has provided more energy, a person may feel totally listless in the absence of the drug.

As with many other areas of physical challenge for the person who dances with chronic illness, the aim is "quality." This means quality of life today and in the future. There is no perfect route to take, no yellow brick road to follow. However, empowering one's self, if one dances with illness, is the key to living well with whatever the outcome or circumstances may be. Experiencing a sense of "this is my educated choice for today" renders contentment and makes living with chronic illness much easier.

We are fortunate to live in times when pharmacists and physicians are demystified to the point where we can, as patients, communicate with them on an even footing. It needs to be a partnership – and it *can* be, once we have done our homework as they have done theirs, and once we are knowledgeable about what is happening to our bodies and about what will be the best way to treat the situation.

Drugs, Drugs and More Drugs

from Sarah's diary

My teenaged son was alarmed last night when he opened the drawer in my nightstand; he noticed the many bottles of pills that I use or have used. It was his consternation that made me think about my situation with all this medication. Honestly, I had not realized it fully; I have probably been too drugged.

In the morning, I ache so much in the joints that I need a painkiller. Once I can move a bit, it's time for my antidepressant, followed by my antibiotic which I've been on since my pancreatitis attack. Next comes my oral steroid, followed by the medication for ulcer which I have as a result of the steroids. Of course, I need something to sleep because the steroid really wires me up! When did I become such a pill taker? It seems that every little thing that I report to my doctor requires a new medication.

When I tried to slack off on the sleeping pills, I was up all night. The next day, I dragged around so bad that I decided that sleep was more important; I don't remember sleeping without the medication. To tell you the truth, I think that I am addicted to the false sense of well-being that comes from my steroid; it's great, almost like a permanent high.

If I speak to my doctor about this, he might realize just how much I actually take and cut me off. Then what will I do?

Drug abuse and addiction are also common with the life of chronically ill persons. Many symptoms are managed through chemical treatment and the sufferer is not always the one to blame. It is a sad fact that not all physicians keep close tabs on exactly how much and which medications their patients are actually taking. It is very easy for the challenged to fall into the trap because escape – from pain, from insomnia and other discomforts – is a natural thing to seek out.

Chronic means forever. Because of this sentence to "life" with a chronic challenge, symptom management through natural ways is recommended to avoid addiction. For the pain and stiffness of the morning, what about a warm shower or a gentle massage from a caregiver? Would hot milk, less caffeine and sugar, be good alternatives to sleeping medication? Is a steroid treatment always necessary? Could one avoid infection by using more natural soaps?

When one deals with a chronic state, it is imperative to remember just what chronic means: forever. So, if at the age of 40, a person is challenged, then they must meet the challenge the rest of their life. This is the main reason for being as free from medication as possible. There are natural herbs and natural ways in which one can manage their symptoms. Chemical treatments can best be taken when there is really no other alternative. In this event, the challenged are wise to become familiar with the make-up of what they are ingesting and its side effects so as to manage their treatment properly.

Drug addiction becomes the second chronic challenge for the chronically ill. This is a sad reality that one must face and deal with as soon as possible. Because chronic illness is the perfect place for addiction, when all drugs are readily available and masked under the disguise of treatment, one needs to develop an astuteness with regards to their chemical intake.

Have Chair Will Travel

from Sarah's diary

Once David pushed me into the video store, I let him know that I needed to wheel myself around solo. The carpet made the wheeling difficult; this only added to the realization that this manual wheelchair is a relic.

This was a trial run, I won't purchase one of my own at present. This loaner should give me the opportunity to experiment.

How difficult will it be for David to push me around? I'm pretty heavy; will he be able to do it? Do we plan ahead, check out the ramps, before going out with it? What if we run into my sister or one of our friends?

How will David and the kids experience this emotionally? What will it feel like to sit in one of these? Am I ready for this darn thing?

This is so much more than simply a "mobility aid." There was so much more to this journey this morning. How I wish I had broken a leg instead of having been diagnosed with lupus. David practices pushing me around; he experiments with backing down bumps and into entrances, walking with his back straight and reacting to my "stop" and "watch that person's feet."

It was great to be able to choose for myself the videos that interest me and since my knees just hurt too much to walk this morning, the chair helped. I sat in the chair while David paid and I thought: "Now that wasn't so bad..."

I am really aching today and thankful for this symbol of "disability" that actually gives me "ability" to get out.

After reading Sarah's entry, we probably agree that she is dancing superbly well with her condition. She seems willing to fight relentlessly, even if she waits until things become too uncomfortable and force her to change. Probably her parents did a good job of giving her the opportunity to develop her "never say die" attitude. She deserves praise for her determination to get out into the world even if it means that she must accommodate her disease with the use of a wheelchair. It takes time and a certain amount of fine tuning before one gets to the place where we know just when to push the reset button. Attitudes, expectations and emotions may need to alter before we feel ready to move on.

This is the whole difference between giving in to the illness and learning to dance with it. Our illness presents limitations, that is a certainty. Often, if we can change the focus, alter the way in which we do such and such, change the place where we are active, use proper time and symptom management, we can live our lives as we decide. In effect, the chronic illness tags along, but the person affected takes the lead in the dance.

At the request of the physician, the physiotherapist or occupational therapist will work with the patient to select the right equipment for mobility. Since a great deal of time might be spent in this chair, the owner wants to ensure that no unwanted side effects, such as sores or back trouble, will be generated from an inadequately fitting chair. The cost of such a vehicle is high; many agencies, societies, and certain government programs can help in the funding. Patients need to go through the correct channels, beginning with their family physician, in order to acquire the available funding to purchase their wheelchair.

There are proper techniques to use when pushing a manual wheelchair; it is not simply a matter of pushing. For the person sitting in the chair, the experience can be terrifying if the attendant does not know how to properly maneuver the vehicle. Many bumps are better taken backwards. The patient's feet extend outward so the pusher must be careful not to run into anyone. The brakes are the safety which keep the patient from flying off their horse. It is a good idea for the attendant to take a turn sitting in the chair and to experience being pushed around. This will help the caregiver get in touch with the experience of the one sitting in the chair. The key is to never take for granted that you know how they must feel until you have had a taste of it. Like any other new skill, pushing a wheelchair or driving one is something that one practices in order to become effective.

For a chronically ill person, being initiated and becoming comfortable with a wheelchair is a long and painstaking journey. Although we have focused on the physical element of using a wheelchair, its emotional challenge is of great significance and will be discussed in a later chapter. A person using a wheelchair as a mobility aid would do well to establish a relationship with this new challenge; with the chair, one gains an *ability* and isn't that what dancing with chronic illness is all about?

Caring for the Ill Parts
from Leah's diary

Today I picked up my fifth pair of designer glasses in the last two years. Sometimes I think I've become self-indulgent, but then I think how all of these glasses are emotionally therapeutical and physically necessary.

The practice of keeping in fashion as well as abreast of new thinner types of lenses are my ways of coping with the visual problems I have because of my MS. After 22 years of wearing contact lenses, I felt ugly in glasses. I was back to the "Coke bottle" look. The day I lost sight in my left eye is the day I lost my ability to wear contacts. I'll never forget that day. I decided there was no way I was going to live with ugly, ordinary glasses.

I have Christian Dior glasses for going out on the town; Jessie Raphael glasses for working around the house; fancy pinkish coral glasses for the soft feminine days; and the cool prescription shades for driving and for the days when my eyes burn. The second pair of Jessie Raphael glasses I wear exclusively for reading.

My disease may win some battles during its life, but I am winning the war.

In effect, what Leah has done is adorn the challenged part of her body; her eyes are attacked and so she enhances them, cares for them, having learned to love them even when they are ill. This a perfect example of effectively grieving a loss through physical challenge due to chronic illness. Rather than a rejection, there is an acceptance of the physical limitation. Any rejection of any part of one's body adds to the unhealthiness of that part. Proper grieving allows acceptance through the nurturing of the challenged part and will create a peaceful living "with" the limitation. In some cases, the affected parts of the body have actually healed. If the challenged person can come to love and accept their physical dimension, regardless of its limitations, it is safe to assume that their dance with illness will be eased.

It can be hard work to come to feel this way about one's challenged body. We must realize that much of this hinges on the "before" situation of the challenged person. When body image has been a thorn in one's side prior to illness, then after the onset of chronic illness one's body image will not improve; in fact, it will likely worsen. What once was a less than acceptable *body image* now becomes an *unacceptable body*. Keep in mind that chronic illness does not change the essence of who a person really is, but it might worsen the situation for the challenged person.

Rather than rejecting our ill body, running away at the sight of our suffering body, we must embrace it. Only then, even with the possibility of further degeneration, do we have a chance to live in peace with our body.

More or Less Accessible
from Leah's diary

It looks like I won't be going to that movie theater anymore. I gave my hubby an earful. "Shit! There's snow all over the parking sign on the pavement...a lot of help that is. Why in hell don't these yo-yo's put up a sign on a post? We only get an average of five feet of snow during the winter! If I try to walk in from a regular spot, the distance to walk will do me in for the night."

Of course, someone without a handicapped decal took it, not realizing it was designated. When we finally got into the building, I gave my hubby another earful. "Oh God, there are over 30 steps to the washroom; I can't handle this...you know that I piddle at least three times during the movie. By the time I get up those stairs, I'll need 9-1-1."

I wanted to cry. We had to leave. Jeff wanted to speak to the manager so that I could use the facility in his office, but I did not want to create a scene.

This is my lot in life now; I just have to live with these things. I guess it's not so bad, I can always rent a video.

Everyone knows that watching *Mr. Holland's Opus* on a television screen just doesn't bring out the music like the big screen does. Even if the popcorn is fresh, watching *Jurassic Park* on the tube just doesn't cut it. Why should Leah not enjoy the same entertainment as any other citizen? She is definitely giving up where she could do something about the situation. Leah must not allow her fears and her "I don't want to create a fuss attitude" to sabotage her real needs.

Accessibility is the law. However, the quality and the effectiveness of that accessibility is not always consistent. Some ramps are suicide paths for a wheelchair because of their degree of incline. Some parking spots have the sign on the pavement, which is of little use if you live in an area with snowy winters. Then, some of the designated spots are not wide and so you cannot get a wheelchair properly set up beside the vehicle.

Not all public places abide by the laws. Instead of suffering in silence, the challenged can use their voices to shout out the injustice. Sometimes, proprietors simply need to be educated about what effective accessibility really is. Some public domains need lobbying before they actually spend the money to make public spaces accessible.

Even when we are considered loud-mouthed activists, we can be certain of our responsibility to ourselves and to our fellow "in-mates" to raise issues for our rights and our quality of life. By being victims, silent sufferers, we help no one; it is through us, the challenged, that the world wakes up and learns of our needs. We must DO something.

Coping with "Handicapped" Parking

from Sarah's diary

I could have hit that "so and so" for having the audacity to ask me why I was parking in the handicapped space. He apologetically responded that he had not noticed my decal. What really got to me is when he said, "You don't look handicapped, lady." How ignorant! How totally ignorant! You can be sure I let him have it, and said, "I think you're the crippled one, you asshole!" Then I mouthed off about how some of us are plagued with illnesses that nobody sees. This damn condition. At least if I had something with stuff that people could notice, they wouldn't look at me as if I am a fat lazy cow! I'd like to slice off all this fat so that this damned disease could show through! I look like an overgrown balloon! Some parking hell this city is!

Sarah is having a terrible time. The parking incident propels her anger into rage. It takes a certain amount of time and experience for a person with a challenge to become comfortable with parking in handicapped spaces. Sometimes one may feel guilt if they are having a good day. Of course, along with the spatial dimension is the harsh realization that you have inherited a visual label. There are always those who speak too quickly and before they engage their mind they have already questioned your need for a handicapped spot. When the signs are on the pavement and winter sets in, it becomes a guessing game. When the spaces are not designed properly, you fight to remove your wheelchair from your vehicle. Not all designated parking spots actually provide an easier access into buildings.

Challenged persons need to take time to stake out a place before parking. Whatever the passengers or the other drivers think of one's decision to park in a designated spot is irrelevant. It is important to care for oneself or, in some cases, to defend oneself from the rest of the world. When an empathic stranger lends you a hand or a smile, you can add to your belief in the goodness of humanity.

We should never pass judgment on whether or not a person is challenged. For every visible impairment there is an invisible one. The mere fact that a car has a designated decal should be enough for us to respect that situation. It is a well-known truth that some persons take advantage; the teenager who takes grandma's decal to go to the mall is in effect cheating the system. Let's leave it to that teen to work out the dilemma within their own conscience. Our role is to empower the challenged, to support them in their endeavor to lead a quality life. If situations arise where we think people need to be educated about building codes and accessibility, we can inform them politely of our concern and even direct them to get the relevant literature. Sometimes they will be grateful, and sometimes not. We offer the education and leave the outcome to them.

Is handicapped parking a privilege for the challenged? No, there is no such thing as a privilege in the world of chronic illness. Handicapped parking is a form of parking that best suits the needs of the challenged. Let's get the word out to ourselves and to those who are not chronically challenged.

Don't Touch My Stuff

from Bob's diary

I could have killed Marcia this morning. Because sometimes she doesn't listen or care where she leaves her stuff, I could not find my glasses. After struggling to get up and look for them, I was so exhausted that I had to lie down again. I was too angry to sleep. You'd think that after nine years of my wrestling with chronic fatigue she would know that it's rough for me to sit and live in this damned recliner. I hate Marcia for being the way she is, I hate this damned disease for making me feel like a cripple and I hate the invalid I have become. It's not too much to ask that she leave my stuff alone; everything I need is there, in its place where I can get to it without trouble. Doesn't she think of that at all?

Bob's concerns which might appear as pettiness to an able-bodied person are legitimate to a challenged person. The physical environment takes on this great importance since it is still within the ill person's control, not to mention the fact that it makes life much easier for the person. So many of the small tasks and movements that well persons take for granted – for example, getting up to get a misplaced pair of reading glasses – can become an exhausting activity for a person suffering from chronic fatigue.

In their homes or in their hospital rooms, patients arrange their nests. The telephone is within reach, the window blind is adjusted to the desired amount of light, the clock is sitting where it can be seen from a lying position. This is how we claim our boundaries, how we meet the demands of our limitations. Once again, clear and effective communication is the only way to eradicate flare-ups between the challenged and their caregivers. It is the responsibility of the challenged person to voice their needs appropriately, before rage festers and erupts, causing more pain for both the patient and the loving caregiver.

What Sex Life!

from Sarah's diary

As if I didn't have enough to cope with already, now I've lost my sex drive. It is a part of our relationship that David and I really enjoy and now I just can't get into it. If I didn't know better, I'd say that something has zapped all sexual desire out of me. Forcing myself to engage in it with David was unproductive; I could not even lubricate and the whole ordeal was physically painful.

David is supportive, yet, I feel his frustration with this situation. Often, he begins to caress me when we get into bed, and with each touch I just shiver and don't want to be touched. I am repulsed by any sexual advances that he makes. When I spoke to my doctor about my dry spell, he didn't seem to have any definite answers. I was discouraged at hearing, "Maybe it's a consequence of depression, maybe it's the illness attacking the genitalia, maybe it's the beginning of menopause..." His list of "maybes" discouraged me and reaffirmed that the joys of sexual pleasure have been robbed from my relationship. We were so close when we were sexual, so good at it.

The other night, I experimented with alcohol. The only result was exhaustion and yearning to sleep. It is so pathetic for me to see myself reduced to this asexual state.

A loss of sex drive and overall interest in sex can be direct results of physical challenge through a chronic illness. It matters little whether the problem is numbness, pain or repulsion. What is real is the loss of an area of one's life that strengthens self-confidence and enhances the relationship with one's self and one's partner.

With some challenged persons as well as for their partners who take care of them, the mere physical exhaustion brought on by dancing with chronic illness is all it takes to lose sex drive. We cannot neglect the depression stages that are so prevalent in chronic illness, whether they reflect organic depression or situational depression. The manifestations are painful and most often decrease sexual appetite. To further the already difficult situation, some antidepressants cause diminished or lost sex drive as a common side effect. It becomes a vicious circle. Within that whirlwind, we may not want sexual intimacy, we may seek the emotional bonding that is created with sexual connectedness, or we may be rejected by our partner who still wants an active sexual relationship.

Open and effective communication, listening clearly and talking clearly, is the best possible outlet for someone suffering from loss of sex life. Whether with one's partner or with one's physician, the challenged person needs to make an effort to clearly verbalize their suffering with regards to this loss of sexual identity. When a chronically ill person feels like an inadequate sex partner, it is best for them to get that fear out in the open. The partner who no longer sees the challenged person as a desirable sexual partner is in their own way challenged emotionally and in need of support and help.

If the situation leads to infidelity on the part of the non-challenged partner, the reality is that the relationship had weak intimacy and commitment before the onset of chronic illness; the disease becomes the excuse for unfaithfulness. A healthy, loving relationship can endure a loss of sexual activity, whether it be intermittent or permanent. Chronically ill persons and their partners need to learn the fine nuances of their dance with illness.

As with all other counterparts of physical challenge, this one entails an emotional challenge. We will discuss the emotional dimension further in chapter four, even though we realize that both dimensions are most often intertwined. The chronically ill person is a target for a multitude of physical losses, adaptations and changes; it takes considerable time and, most of all, much emotional energy to meet the overall challenge of chronic illness. The chronically ill person needs to examine their sexual life to become aware of how it differs from before the onset of the illness. What does differ is the way in which the sexual dance takes place their life.

This Is So Embarrassing
from Leah's diary

I must have caught a flu bug or something; the evening started out with me throwing up my dinner. Then to make matters worse, as I was vomiting, my bladder gave out and I wet myself. What a sight! In the bathroom, with my head in the toilet bowl, my night clothes urine soaked. I felt at my lowest. When I burst into tears, Jeff came in to help me. He reassured me that it was the violent vomiting that brought on the incontinence. He kept repeating that this would not be permanent. As he helped me to undress and get into the tub, I caught a glimpse of myself in the vanity mirror. I was crushed, beaten, so very weak and vulnerable. This morning, I managed to get up first so that I could make Jeff his favorite breakfast.

This type of demeaning and horrific episode is one that is too often the reality with which the challenged live. We take certain bodily functions for granted. When debilitating illness strikes a blow, it reduces us to a childlike state. Incontinence is cruel. It conjures up all sorts of old tapes given by our parents when we were toilet trained. Incontinence is punctuated by images of our excretory system being "dirty."

Incontinence targets a person's vulnerability and self-esteem, as well as healthy sexuality. The caregiver reduces the impact with comforting words, reminding them that "this is just an accident, something that will pass." If we are not fortunate in having such a compassionate partner, then we need, for our own survival, to give ourselves those positive messages. Looking at ourselves in the mirror at this precise time is not the best way to go. We would be more nurtured by holding on to ourselves, by giving ourselves a hug. As soon as possible, we should resume our lives with some sort of routine activity that brings us joy.

Time on My Hands

from Bob's diary

Marcia got on my case for watching too much television. What the hell else am I supposed to do? If she only understood that I don't necessarily like to watch TV all day, but I have so much damned time on my hands. Before I got sick, I watched the daily news and the odd game on the tube. Now, as soon as I get up in the morning, within 30 minutes I have done everything that I have to do. The rest of the day drags on forever. Reading is no good because I can't concentrate to follow the damn story; anyway I'm too depressed to read. I couldn't care less. At least with television, I can just sit there. All of a sudden I'm riding a Harley with Schwartzenegger or fighting bad guys with Pacino. What does Marcia expect me to do if I don't watch TV? Lately, even those awful soap operas interest me. I know my brain is turning to mush!

Time, a lot of idle time has the potential to destroy mental health. The onslaught of a chronic illness parachutes a person into early retirement. When a person can maintain partial employment, that is the best scenario. But let's focus on a situation like Bob's who is not able to work.

Each day offers a seemingly eternal amount of time. Meanwhile, Bob's mind is not growing and his morale is surely not uplifted. He has no sense of personal achievement or self-esteem in watching other people live their lives while he stands on the sidelines and his own life disintegrates to nothingness. Hobbies can be expensive and there is often the added problem of financial stress.

If financial resources are scarce because of loss of employment, if no disability insurance kicks in, a person with a challenge must work harder to seek meaningful activities to fill their day. Keep a daily calendar of activities, even if the entries are as simple as 7:00 a.m. shower and dress, 8:00

a.m. breakfast, 8:30 a.m. letter writing, etc... This scheduled day provides a person with a sense of accomplishment, the antidote to uselessness. Why not write letters, renew friendships, make lunch dates, organize picture albums or your family history.

Volunteer activities can be extremely rewarding. It is important to volunteer for activities we feel attracted to, maybe the type of thing we have always wished we could do for employment. Of course, voluntarism should never exceed the amount of available time, keeping in mind our energy levels as well. Only a few minutes a day, or a few hours a week is all it takes. Whether we physically get out to do this work or whether we do it from our home is irrelevant. What matters is that we begin to associate ourselves with the idea of being in some way productive again.

Remember, your life isn't over until you say so.

Some chronically ill individuals can discover new avenues which allow them to re-enter the workplace. Before a person gives up entirely on their productivity and allows empty time to corrode their self-esteem, they should investigate the possibilities of rehabilitation. It is not uncommon to learn of persons afflicted with chronic illness who become residents of chronic wards once they stop being productive altogether. We want to ward off that syndrome as long as possible. Whether through government agencies or local social agencies, we can explore other means of "work" within the limitations we have.

Fear keeps a person from going out into the world accompanied by chronic illness. It is an unknown territory, made more intimidating by the new vulnerability that one experiences with the onset of chronic illness.

Sometimes the challenged live with old tapes that cast them in certain types of work with seemingly no other alternatives. It is time for challenged persons to dig deeper into the reasons why they fear certain areas of productivity and to go into battle against these imaginary demons. There is more time and opportunity for many challenged persons to further their formal education after a diagnosis. We can be productive and fulfilled from a chair or from a bed if need be. *The only limits are those we put on ourselves.* It is in taming of disease, accommodating the disease, and developing our personal dance step, that we live: first, fully, and second, with a disease. Bob can be a productive and fulfilled man who just happens to dance with a chronic illness.

Could You Cut My Meat Please?
from Sarah's diary

What an eye opener at lunch yesterday! I ordered my meal, not realizing that the roast turkey would require cutting; my plate sat in front of me as I grappled with my good arm and hand, trying to cut a piece off with my fork. I was frustrated. Pat just sat there, perfectly calm, eating away, not even noticing my struggle. I was hungry after 10 minutes of the struggle.

All of a sudden, it hit me; of course, it was up to me to ask for help. Once I did, she immediately cut my food and added, "I was wondering when you would ask." She is a great friend, who respects me as a person, who never imposes any limitations that I do not first acknowledge. I learned a good lesson: it's up to me how people will treat me and it's up to me to get what I need.

Challenged persons must ask for what they need. People around us do not know when and how to ask if we need assistance. They fear we may be offended if they cater to us before we ask. Everything we can do, we should do. We should ask for assistance to accomplish what is impossible or too difficult. It is a simple matter of taking our power of choice and using it.

Sarah had to be ready emotionally for someone cutting her food for her. Pat would have humiliated Sarah had she taken charge of the cutting too soon. Sarah had to figure out her needs and then ask for assistance. At first, some challenged persons experience that as demeaning, which it can be. As time goes by and after needless frustration, we learn that others are more than willing to help us; we can give them a sense of worth by accepting their help.

At the same time, we want to guard against becoming over dependent on others. When do we really need help and when do we simply want attention? I am reminded of a paraplegic man who suffered from severe loneliness; he would ask his little girl to bring him some water so that he could cajole her and have some company for a few minutes. If we need affection, we must ask for it. Once again, we must use our reasonable mind to determine whether we are overdoing it to the extent of pushing away those we love most.

As in all areas of life, one must learn to communicate effectively with oneself first, and then with the world around. Straight communication is the key to a healthy relationship in all its dimensions. Whether we need to have a steak cut up, a glass of water brought to our bedside, or our bottoms wiped after a bowel movement, all needs are the responsibility of the one afflicted. We take the lead in the two-step with the challenge...always.

Home Sweet Home

from Leah's diary

More and more I don't go down to the family room in the evening; the stairs just wipe me out. When we bought our house, there was no evidence of any chronic illness for me. The plan we chose has three different levels, which were a breeze back then. Now, with my left leg dragging, my back sore from using the cane, and the exhaustion brought on by my last attack, I struggle to get around. Sometimes just contemplating going up the five steps to my bedroom is exhausting. My evenings, in my bedroom, are lonely; I hear my family laughing at a television sitcom or my two teenagers arguing over homework. I feel cut off from them.

Yesterday I tried to cook dinner and to stand on my feet for a while. I have to stand because if I sit down to cook, the counters are way too high. The kitchen was designed for a woman of average energy, who could stand on her two feet. My daughter pitched in and finished preparing what I had started, so we did have dinner.

Taking my shower is becoming frightening because I tend to get very weak under the hot water. I have not told anyone in my family, but I usually take my shower early in the evening because I am afraid to do it when they are out or in bed. At least, if I do it early, I know they are around.

What is happening is that our house just is not appropriate for me anymore and my doctor has not shown optimism about my getting better; this chronic problem is here to stay. What do I do? The kids and Jeff adore this home. I am attached to my home and I sure as heck have lost enough already without losing my nest.

What Leah is living through is typical of the stress that arises acutely or progressively when a home is not adapted to the needs of a chronically challenged person. Moving from one room to the other, while presenting no problem to the able-bodied, is a feat for the challenged. Persons may isolate themselves in the areas where they can get around without strain. They may even add to their physical symptoms or problems by overdoing it because the house is just not adapted. Narrow doorways create havoc for wheelchairs, kitchen counters are too high for a person sitting to cook and cupboards are similarly out of reach for the challenged cook.

A kitchen is a primary room in a home; the counters must be lowered to accommodate a person sitting while cooking; so must a stove, an oven, a dishwasher and any other kitchen appliances. If the house has levels, then a one-person lift may take care of the stairs problem.

There are plans to follow and building information is available from medical stores or from government agencies. The washroom should be equipped with bars in the tub, also a lowered vanity and sink, and any other medical aid that the challenged may need. With many challenged persons, an air conditioned environment in the summer is no luxury. Some associations may assist in the financing of such things and in some jurisdictions the expenses are medical deductions. If the challenged family member needs to use a wheelchair, the ramp outside the home should be built according to specific plans so as to maximize safety and resistance to weather conditions. The whole idea being that the more independent the chronically ill person can be, the better for all concerned.

Home is the best place to be for the challenged person. After a hospital stay, the challenged person will heal and gain back control over their lives more quickly in their own nest. For this reason, a person's home must be adapted to whichever stage they are in. It is not a matter of privilege, it is more a matter of a right to comfort. The challenged family member needs to be able to cook a meal for their family, to watch television in the same room, in effect, to be a full participant in the household without any constraints brought on by poor accessibility.

The onslaught of chronic illness does not have to make one less than Queen or King of the castle.

The physical challenge of chronic illness is usually addressed first. Because its factors are tangible, measurable and visible, treatment follows. The physician prescribes medications; drug treatments are administered and the enlightened patient watches for addiction. A builder adapts the home, the caregiver places things for easy access. The challenged person accepts and learns to use mobility aids, accepts and learns to love the ill parts of their body. The dance is smooth and synchronized, given time and effort. Everyone becomes educated about handicapped parking and accessibility. Their education breaks the barriers of hush-hush topics like sexuality and adaptation to that loss. They tackle the more embarrassing predicaments, like bowel or urine incontinence. Progressively, the challenged person learns that they are responsible for their own care. They claim that responsibility and those around them learn from this awareness.

Of the three dimensions of challenge – physical, emotional and spiritual – the first, the physical, is the most manageable; the dance is choreographed easily enough. But deep in the heart of the person living with chronic illness is the emotional challenge. Here, in isolation, alone with the emotional monsters, the challenged person fights the Great War.

FOUR

The Emotional Challenge

Our Feelings in the Dance

To My Eyes

You gift me with sight
of mountains and lakes and snow,
of my son's smile,
and
of my lover's smirk.

You open up my universe
in the early morning sunshine.
You bring into my home
artists, actors, musicians, dancers.

With you, I travel independently
on country roads and superhighways,
take my son to a baseball game,
and
my lover out for dinner.

But, of all the gifts you bestow,
You, my eyes, are the key to seeing
into another's soul.
If I should lose you
This is what I would grieve the most.

The physical challenges ushered in by chronic illness can be treated either by medication, by physiotherapy, or by natural symptom management techniques. But a person's inner world is an entirely different situation. If the challenged person aspires to take the lead in the dance, then what they feel and what they do with that feeling self, remains their responsibility. This task will undoubtedly be the most difficult ever undertaken. We have already dealt with the grieving cycle in chapter two. Grief presents a whole universe of emotional challenge. In this present chapter, on emotional challenge, we will provide a glimpse into the complex inner emotional world of the chronically challenged.

Because one's actions stem from one's thinking and feeling dimension, the emotional challenge takes on great significance in the dance with chronic illness. If the emotional challenge is dealt with successfully, then the physical challenge can be met with much greater ease.

Part of the complexity of this challenge rests in the unknown; we do not always know what we feel. It takes concentrated effort to come to a place where one can effectively name the exact emotion that is activated inside our heart, then comes the arduous task of dealing with that emotion. As we can well understand, it will take considerable time for us to name the emotion and then to move into claiming that emotion. What do we do with the emotion then?

More often than not, we will need to reprogram or to program for the first time, healthy mental attitudes toward the variety of elements in the emotional challenge of chronic illness. The magnitude of our emotional life itself may have been neglected until now because we have been physically able to produce and to keep busy, *too busy to think or to feel.*

When illness strikes, there is an abundance of "thinking" and "feeling" time, replacing the "producing" time. We face a great challenge. This explains the personality and temperament changes that so often accompany a person who is diagnosed with a chronic illness. *We are who we were*, however, we *do* alter the *way* in which we are; our focus changes.

Chronically ill persons are intensely emotional persons; fatigue and exhaustion, medication and emotional roller coasters brought on by the unpredictability of disease contribute to this emotional fragility. Chronic illness is a "heart" disease in that it attacks our feeling self. Of course, this overwhelming phenomenon affects caregivers in the exact same way.

If the chronically ill person is healthy emotionally, then we will be amazed at their resilience in the face of physical challenge. They will live with a quality of life, in spite of their chronic illness. The emotions they host, because they are emotionally challenged, are neither good, bad, condemnable nor neglectable. They must be faced, named and claimed.

It's Good To Have a Friend

from Sarah's diary

When Mary called, I just about hung up on her. What chutzpah! After not inviting me to her daughter's wedding, she calls me to tell me about it. Before this damn disease, we did everything together. My life is so different now and it makes me angry as hell. She and some other friends are saying that I'm nothing but a volcano ready to erupt. Nobody wants to be around me. My handicap has robbed me of my life; if I could make somebody pay for this, I sure as hell would.

Now, what about the matter of Sarah's anger? It certainly takes on the proportions of rage in this incident. Her chronic illness has interfered considerably with her friendship with Mary, with whom she *did* a lot of things. Sarah, at present, is *doing* things very differently than before. For some reason neither Mary nor Sarah have *talked* and *listened* around the issue of how the disease affects them both. I suspect that Mary is uncertain about how and when to strike up a conversation about this issue; if Sarah is oozing this anger everywhere, then Mary will certainly not bring up any potentially difficult topics. It is Sarah's responsibility to strike up the tune.

Sarah wants to make somebody pay; she is looking for a target – an absolutely normal reaction in these circumstances. It's unhealthy that Mary is the target for now; tomorrow, someone else will be the target. If Sarah begins to place herself in the position of the target, then her rage can be potentially dangerous; it can reach suicidal dimensions.

Anger is an energizing emotion; it is also a secondary emotion. One needs to go to the source, to the first emotion – in this case, great sadness and possibly fear. Sarah can expect to do a lot of crying, seeking comfort during this naming and claiming of the sadness of life as she has known it. Following some resolution of the primary emotion, Sarah needs to learn how to use her anger effectively, creatively, and to her advantage. Proper anger management can include:

- seeking professional therapy if I feel stuck in the anger
- giving careful consideration to whom I ask for help
- verbalizing my anger and raging words
- drawing a picture of my target, giving it the anger
- pounding a pillow or other safe surface
- writing an angry letter and then tearing it up
- giving myself permission to cry
- protecting myself from hooking into others' anger
- setting limits for time when I vent my anger
- using my anger as energy.

Within the world of the chronically challenged, friendships are kept alive or born in the same way as they are in the unchallenged world. We are fooled into thinking that everything changes when chronic illness hits. Not so, and it need not be so where our friends are concerned. Healthy and effective communication is mandatory for everyone concerned.

For many people with chronic illness, friendships change. We do not need to lose our unchallenged friends; it is however, our responsibility to educate them so that they can consider our limitations. If we become an angry person, chances are that we will lose our friends. This is not because we are challenged, but because we are angry. Focusing away from the challenged world is healthy since it encourages us to reinstate ourselves as "normal" citizens who happen to be challenged rather than continue only as victims of illness. We must maintain a well-rounded life within the challenged circle and outside of it.

At the onslaught of chronic illness, our close friends will not know how to be with us. It is the "what do I say, what do I do" syndrome. They are saddened and most feel helpless to assist. Many simply stay away rather than face the sadness our presence triggers. A woman bumps into an old friend, now in a wheelchair, "You know, I saw you in the emergency room about two years ago; I could not bring myself to talk to you...just seeing you in the chair...I was a coward..." The challenged woman replies, "It hurt too much, hey?"

The specter of chronic illness knows no bounds; its helter-skelter character targets anyone. Part of the emotional difficulty people have relating to a friend, once they are diagnosed with chronic illness, is fear of their own mortality. If it can happen to her, than it could happen to me. Life is fragile and as much as we may fool ourselves into thinking otherwise, hangs by a thread. The chronically challenged person symbolizes the power of the beast within chronic illness. This explains the uneasiness and even the disdain that certain persons experience when they are in the presence of a challenged person; *they see only the disease and not the person.*

We need to evaluate the impact of our friendships at intervals; are they taking more away from us than we can afford emotionally? On what are our friendships based? Office relationships, for example, probably will not survive the end of one's career and that is simply logical. There is value in making new friends among those that live with chronic illness although here, we must remain cautious that our lives do not become filled solely with illness and its victims. Our relationships with others who suffer the same types of woes are gifts indeed, as are our relationships outside that circle that keep us actively involved in all types of lifestyles.

Incarceration at the Big H
from Leah's diary

Well, here I am again, in bed 2, room 215. I cried all night long; when the nurse came in to ask what was wrong, I told her everything was all right. I thought she was too busy to sit with me for a while. This is my third bout in hospital this year. Actually it's not so bad; sometimes I think I'm spoiled. The food is something I have grown to almost enjoy; the small portions help my weight problem. My sister wanted to come to visit but I told her not to bother since she is busy. If only I can find ways to occupy my time. So far, I don't feel like doing anything.

If the nurses were not so occupied, I would have called one, but I waited. My drip was going too quickly. It hurt like hell! Last time, when I was here, I found that crying a lot made me sleepy; hopefully, I'll exhaust myself crying again and fall asleep. Maybe this will all be a dream when I wake up.

In this entry, Leah discounts her own needs while she assumes that others have more important needs. This type of attitude will be discussed further in the book as one possible position that we take in relationship to others.

The experience of hospitalization requires adjustment and tolerance. When chronic illness is a life sentence, the person so sentenced can expect to serve some, and perhaps much, of their "time" in hospital. However, the condemned need not lay down and cry for the rest of their hospital stays. Many creative persons discover ways to cope with the reality of these places, where they are *sometimes treated as a disease and not like a person.* In some instances, the challenged person is relieved to be hospitalized while at other times the stay is difficult.

Usually it takes a while before a positive attitude clicks into gear and we accept our incarceration without losing the dignity of our quality of life. The sooner we go through the anger and the depression often associated with hospitalization, the sooner we become healthily accepting of the prison term. Our experience of being hospitalized becomes more livable when we engage in a partnership with the staff. If we validate their caring efforts and recognize their legitimate and frustrated positions, we join them in partnership against the disease.

The power of choice, the most important asset a chronically ill person can hold on to, must be maintained in a hospital setting. While respecting the limitations of the staff and a general running of the hospital, a patient can still make decisions and have choices. Filling a menu, choosing the color of a nightshirt, answering a phone call, seeing a visitor and many other small activities should be the choice of the person afflicted. The empowerment that the patient feels translates positively into their general medical condition and brings a sense of participation.

The very tiny eight foot by ten foot cubicle, around which the bed curtain wraps, is home for the patient for the term of the hospitalization. In this nest, the person sleeps, eats, thinks, reads, exercises if they can, and possibly has intimate conversations. How then can one justify not knocking when entering, or nonchalantly opening the curtain as they walk by? Where is the respect of space for the patient? Would the same person who unthinkingly opens the curtain without asking permission, walk into the patient's house without ringing the doorbell? Do caregivers see that little cubicle as the "home" of the patient?

Whoever enters the "home" of the patient should respect the boundaries that the patient has developed. We must raise awareness within the community of caregivers and medical staffs. Because the chronically ill may have difficulty with mobility, the telephone must always be put back in its place, the bed should be adjusted to suit the needs of the patient, whatever items are placed on the night stand should be put back exactly where they were by the cleaning staff, etc.

Patients should be encouraged to have private visitations with their partners. Affectionate or sexual contact might be the best remedy for the isolation felt by a chronically ill person during hospitalization. Can the hospital provide a place and time for these interludes? Some institutions have privacy rooms while others have not even conceived the notion.

Since a hospital stay can be emotionally draining, it is vital to raise awareness of the medical staff to the challenges faced by the patient. Equally important is the knowledge to be learned by the challenged themselves. They need to be educated about the functioning of a hospital, about their limitations or rights, about the social aspect of community living. If the challenged person is a loner, than sharing a room will be difficult if not painful. Whenever the challenged person can express their needs and claim their own power of choice, they become an asset to the nursing staff.

Chronically ill individuals will spend extended periods of time in hospitals. How we cope with our hospital stays has everything to do with how we have grown into the relationship with our dance partner, our disease. As the disease progresses, we will often witness an acclimatization to the unnatural setting of hospital life. Above all, the prescription is quality of life, through taking our power and safeguarding our dignity of choice

Just Like Family
from Sarah's diary

My brother has not called me in six months, not even when David let him know that I was in the hospital last summer. I guess I know who my friends really are. In all honesty, I think that he has a harder time with my illness than I do. Ever since I was diagnosed with lupus, it's like I have something catching. When my sister calls me, the only thing she talks about is her daughter's twins. Who really cares! When she says, "How are you?" she really means to say, "You're the same so let me talk about my stuff." David's sister, on the other hand, is so worried and concerned with my illness, that I don't open up to her; she has enough of her own problems and I want to save her the agony of hearing me out. I have decided not to go to the family Christmas dinner since I think that my family would rather not have me there; they will have more fun without me."

Sarah, like Leah in the last diary entry, has adopted a position where she puts more importance on what others feel and do than she puts on her own personal experiences. In the chapter on communication, we will take a closer look at this attitudinal position.

It is not uncommon for family members to be at a loss when one of them is diagnosed with a chronic illness. Some feel guilty because they remain unaffected. Some are naturally frightened by the implied fragility of their own health. Some just were never emotionally close to the one who is diagnosed.

The most effective course of action is for the diagnosed person to take the lead. We need to make the first move, to call the shots, to make that phone call in hopes of expressing just what we are living. Those members who are attuned and sympathetic need to be thanked, not protected. Usually, people know how much they can take and if they are tuned into our pain, it must be because they feel that they can handle it.

It is never a solution to avoid family gatherings; the result is an isolated life away from those we are naturally bonded to. Perhaps some preparation is in order before we go to the gathering, calling each member individually and discussing our apprehensions about the party is an excellent idea. This way, everyone has time to get emotionally ready for the event.

One basic truth remains: *others will treat us as we treat ourselves*. When we are challenged with chronic illness, we influence how others will experience us and the relationship between ourselves and others.

What Night Life?
from Leah's diary

Even after explaining to Jeff that I just don't want to go out at night, he still asks me. Last night he wanted to go out for dinner and I didn't have the courage to go into explanations again, so I gave in. I looked so tired when I glanced in the mirror of the restaurant washroom. This illness has zapped me totally, in such a way that I will never be the same again. Oh well, I guess it's my mother's words haunting me: "We have our crosses to bear."

Jeff means well of course. It is very difficult for him to understand the exhaustion. I love him; put up with my own pain for him.

Any type of emotional and physical expending of energy becomes overwhelming. All those well-meaning "Hello, how are you?" questions when one steps out into the world, can be a suffering in themselves. The honest response is, "Awful...dragging myself around...wish this disease would go away..."

Some chronically ill persons cannot summon the courage to communicate effectively that they are not in a proper condition to go out, especially at night. For the woman who, in her past life, was always made up and perky, finding herself exhausted after uttering a few words is emotionally painful. Going out at night becomes impossible. Her sexuality takes a beating. As a result, she may retreat more and more into her own home because going out is just too taxing. For the man who was a social animal, always joking and bantering back and forth, going out can become very different. He will want to retreat at home where no one questions him about his work, which he probably has abandoned because of illness.

The primary caregiver to the chronically challenged person needs to learn exactly what the boundaries are where going out is concerned. If going out is important to the caregiver, then by all means they should do so. Here the challenged need to develop a sense of understanding and willingness to accept the outings of their caregiver. Often, the care giving can be done by someone else while the primary caregiver goes out, or the challenged person may be capable of being alone for awhile.

Still there is a danger in becoming too homebound, a certain comfortable rut for the challenged person and a frustrating rut for the caregiver. Both parties must develop healthy communication patterns and settle these situations when they come up. Perhaps they need to manage time more effectively, so that the challenged person prepares by resting for the outing. Perhaps the challenged partner needs to assume responsibility for free time for the caregiver. Perhaps the caregiver needs to develop empathy for the stress brought on by socializing.

Kids, These Days!

from Bob's diary

What a sleepless night I had! Jamie didn't come home until two in the morning. Even though I tried to explore that, as a new driver, he should not have been driving during that blizzard last night, he wouldn't listen. I've lost any power

I had over the kids. They think that because I'm sick now, because their mom works to help support us, I'm not able to parent anymore. It doesn't help that I'm depressed most of the time, living most of my life between the couch and the bed. Along with all the other losses, I've lost my place as a father. My kids don't respect me.

Parenting from a perceived weak place is a challenge. This is especially true if the children have experienced the parent's disposition and attitude before and after the onset of chronic illness. As children witness the loss of health, the loss of income, the loss of social life, they will sometimes assume that their parent has lost the mental and emotional strength to discipline, guide or comfort. What adds to the struggle is the reality of the parent's weakened spirit. Unless a conscious effort is made to empower oneself as a chronically challenged person, parenting becomes an added stress. It is easier to just give up.

A key attribute of successful parenting – and this is true for systems whether or not illness dances within them – is the healthy support of the "well" parent. The automatic emotional and psychological response of a spouse who experiences the illness of a partner is to protect, to care for and at times to overfunction. When such a situation occurs, and it easily does, the patient gets lost in the "being cared for" mode. He or she falls prey to dependency. In some cases, the well parent will keep secrets about the kids' activities so as to not create added stress on the challenged partner.

Often the child cannot verbalize or cope effectively with the new situation. Sometimes this is the setting for "acting out." The behavior is a compensation or a management technique for dealing with repressed emotions. We must keep in mind also that the child may be undergoing the normal changes that come with the child's particular age. The adolescent whose parent is diagnosed with an illness is still an adolescent whose acting out or changed behavior may simply be in keeping with his or her life stage.

When attempting to make some logical observation of the family system struggling with chronic illness, we must always keep in mind that *we are who we were.* The patterns in relationship, the way in which the family system administered itself before, the dynamic of the parents toward the children, remain. Granted the illness may change some of the focus; it may bring losses and a need for renegotiation of responsibilities. It is tempting but dangerous to attribute all the stress of the family system to the chronic illness that has become part of that system.

Doctor, Doctor

from Sarah's diary

Since this was my final checkup before Christmas, I came into Dr. Brown's office today, loaded like Santa Claus. For my doctor, I picked up the latest copy of Dr. Siegel's book on treating ill persons. Since Debbie mentioned last week that with her three kids at home she would not have time to bake, I whipped her up a batch of Santa cookies. Betty roared when she opened her present, an award for "Nurse of the year" shaped like a hypodermic needle. Since Shirley always loses her pen, I got her a pen "on a string."

The staff in this office is like family to me, good family that I count on and visit regularly.

For a person with a chronic illness, the doctor's office becomes a second home. It is common and expected for various medical problems to develop within one's life with chronic illness. To become either self-righteous, overbearing, overdependent or a cry-baby with the staff only causes stress in your life. They will not welcome you when you come in and you won't want to be there either.

Of course, the physician/patient relationship plays a major role in the war against chronic illness. The doctor's secretary may prove to be your best ally in many situations. A little praise for the enormous work done or the personal favor rendered encourages and stimulates good rapport with the person. Before seeing the physician, usually you need to connect with the nurse whether it be for blood pressure, for vital signs, or for opening your file. The nurse also should become an ally in fighting beside you. Even the recordkeeper might warrant a thank you since they keep the reports and prepare the letters for you on the doctor's behalf.

The persons working in your physician's office are the chorus line, the back-up team that you can go into combat with. Remember, they are on your side. Even though they may display their own idiosyncrasies, you can learn to accept them for who they are and to appreciate what they can bring into your life.

Planning for Success

from Leah's diary

What's the use in planning anything! I really wanted to go to my niece's wedding, since she is more like a daughter to me. Yesterday, my doctor suggested I go in for a treatment because of my optic neuritis. I feel that I have no choice . After crying and sobbing about how unfair the whole thing really is, I decided to ask Jeff to go to the wedding without me. It's so difficult for me to be in the hospital and to see him as depressed as I am. We talked about the fact that we should never plan or look forward to anything because of the unpredictability of my illness. It's a sad life and it's mine. I feel so helpless to encourage Jeff who is always there for me. It's not fair how I get a lot more help that he does. I sense that Jeff feels very alone.

In Leah's entry, we read about two different problems: the unpredictability of outings for a challenged person and their partner, and the emotional pain endured by that partner during the course of the disease. Although I will discuss the challenge for the caregiver at greater length later in the book, it becomes painfully apparent that Jeff is living his own challenges with MS. Should he initiate conversations that will most likely lead to emotionally charged topics? What would it be like for him to attend the wedding alone? Does Jeff experience his depression as his wife reports it? How does he cope with the unpredictability in their lives? Instead of both partners agonizing in their own corner, as in this case, is there a place where both could find relief from this strain in their relationship? Both feel powerless, sad and most likely frustrated as they protect each other. Perhaps bringing in a third party, whether their doctor, a therapist or a confidant who could be more objective about their situation, could alleviate some of the pressure for both of them.

It is a trap for persons challenged with chronic illness to not plan ahead for trips and special occasions. We need to have a full life, one that entails activities to look forward to. While being realistic about the possibility of cancellation, we need to make plans as if we do not have any illness. If we do not make plans, then we live at the mercy and under the domination of our disease, being either depressed or raging.

I recommend that we let people know about the risk factor when we commit to future activities. At the same time, I think we should commit with the expectation to participate in events. This planning adds spice to our lives as it does to the lives of those in our circle. When we live with chronic illness, we learn to master the fine balancing act between excessive caution and optimistic expectation in planning. Whatever it takes to bring normality to our lives, to put us among the "living," is what we need to seek out.

Being Sick Is Being Poor
from Bob's diary

Yesterday, after I paid the bills, I figured out that we've got a little over $300 to live on for the rest of the month. It's a major drop in income since I have been on disability. When I worked, my bonus alone, on a good month, added up to more than my disability check does now. So much for being the family provider.

It kills me to see Marcia drag herself around after a day's work; before my illness, we could afford for her to stay home, which is what she really loves to do. People say that money isn't everything; well, maybe they need to live through a chronic illness to find out how poor you can actually get.

Financial stress most often accompanies chronic illness. For some people who are fortunate enough to have adequate insurance that guarantees an income, finances can remain constant. However, for a majority of blue-collar workers, disability income is only a fraction of their former income. Disability income presents a challenge in itself, to obtain and to maintain.

It is not uncommon to have to wait months before papers are filled out and medical reports are forwarded. Usually those months, are "income-less," leaving the family with emptied savings accounts. Even when the disability income is established, insurance companies make it a policy to keep close tabs on the status of the insured person. There are horror stories of unexpected visits from insurance personnel and of pressure letters and phone calls designed to constantly evaluate the legitimacy of the claim. For the ill person battling the disease itself, this financial stress can be devastating.

One way to alleviate the pressure on the ill person is to choose an advocate for the patient. Preferably, the chronically ill person chooses someone familiar with the situation who will take charge of all the correspondence, reports and phone calls. The advocate may be a spouse or family member or friend. The whole premise here is to lessen the stress level for the patient, in financial matters. It does not mean that the ill person is kept in the dark; rather, it means that they are empowered by their advocate. In some cases, a lawyer might be warranted where there is evidence of negligence by the insurance company.

If at all possible, the ill person's partner will take charge of the finances in the system. This is again to minimize the stress to the patient as much as possible. It is amazing how illness renders one vulnerable and emotionally fragile.

How then can the chronically challenged person participate in a healthy way with the finances? A good beginning would be to re-assess your vocational resources and aptitudes. Participating in a vocational rehabilitation program might yield new avenues of productivity. Finding a new line of work through rehabilitation is the best possible way of coping effectively with one's chronic illness. Too much empty time leads to depression and to the downfall of the challenged person's mental health. In the matter of financial stress as in all matters brought about by the onset of chronic illness, you need to take time to re-assess before you make any major decisions concerning your career or your life-style. Giving up too quickly can do more harm than good, and burning yourself out when it's time to let go is equally dangerous.

I Care

from Leah's diary

My whole world crumbled down on me this morning; before I even knew it, Jeff stormed out to go to work. What sticks in my mind is when he raged, "I never do enough and whatever I do is never right!"

Since my diagnosis, he has been my primary caregiver; usually, he doesn't complain when I ask for what I need. For the last few weeks, I have found him very withdrawn, not making much conversation. Sometimes, he rolls his eyes when I ask him to lift my legs and wrap them up with a blanket. I've been too frightened to bring up the subject, but I think that he is fed up with taking care of me.

At times, I want to yell at him that he is negligent and uncaring. Other times, I want to reach out to him and make love to him. And then there are times when I want to release him, to ask him to leave and to make a new life for himself.

Our relationship is different since I am ill. Is he my caregiver now? If so, what happened to my husband? Because I can do so little with him, are we still partners?

I have a terror of becoming a statistic of the marriage breakdown that occurs so often with chronic illness.

Sadly we often focus on the victim and neglect the caregiver. Since I have played the role of a caregiver to my parents, as well as the role of victim of MS, it has become clear to me that care giving causes intense suffering just as does the malady. In the pain of care giving, we experience helplessness, the inability to cease the suffering of those we love and cherish. As a silent witness we are not engaged in the strength of the one who is directly attacked. It is that feeling of impotence that generates suffering from a caregiver's point of view.

There is something powerful for the victim who is connected with her caregiver at the time of pain. It is a sense of shared suffering, of togetherness in the midst of the doom. This sharing is at the heart of what it means to deliver aid: *not to take away the suffering, but to attend to the challenge to walk the road, beside and not for them.*

Just as it takes time for the challenged person to feel empowered to ask for help, it takes some adjustment to the situation before a caregiver realizes that they need assistance and can ask for help. This highlights the importance of community for those struggling with chronic illness. The idea that it's "you and me against the world (or the illness)," is absolutely false, inherently too limited and inevitably destructive. People need to have or to develop a much larger network of support. Caregivers often need as much external support to survive as do the challenged partners. It is amazing and yet common for friends, family or community members to jump in to help in any way they can. Other persons can fill in the gaps when a caregiver has reached their limits.

The primary caregiver must be encouraged to seek out whatever emotional supports *they* need to continue to function; this may include pursuing favorite activities with friends or family, professional counseling, or whatever it takes to restore their own emotional, physical and spiritual health.

Acceptance
from Bob's diary

Marcia is on my case again ever since I stopped meeting the guys for poker on Wednesday nights. She says, "Bob, you're turning into a vegetable...a lonely one..." What really gets me peeved is that I can't stay up long enough at night to play with the guys. By about 8:00, I'm wiped out. Sometimes, I can't even read at night. I tried these energizer-type vitamins and when I told my doctor he freaked out on me. "You have to accept it," he said. Accept what? That my life is over? That I'm nothing more than a has-been? I can't be a provider for my family, I can't stay up at night to meet with my "old" friends...I just can't live with this. As far as I'm concerned, accepting would be giving up. Well, that's not a bad idea at all.

The concept of acceptance takes a considerable amount of time for a person to grasp and much more time to actually experience. Bob is not yet able to accept his limitations and to dance in rhythm with them. When his fatigue gets in the way of socializing he simply gives up that part of his life; his disease has won. Of course, the outcome is that Bob feels less than a person. He fights hard against this fatigue with extra vitamins; when he is not successful, he becomes even more irritable and the disease wins again. No wonder Bob feels beaten.

Acceptance comes after we have learned all about our limitations. Then, it is time to manage our time and our energy, in effect to manage each minute of our living experience. Would a nap before the poker game make it possible for Bob to be part of the gang? Has he considered finding or getting together a group that could meet at a better time? Bob needs to figure out ways of dancing with his limitations without losing those parts of his life that mean a lot to him. When he reaches that point, he will be living in acceptance – not as a loser in the war against his illness, but in partnership with his illness.

Sometimes we think of acceptance in the imagery of calm waters. We need to remember that before this calm came a storm. We must resign ourselves to taking the time to tame the limitations, to working with them, and to learning life management as never before. Active participation, not resignation, is necessary in order to reach acceptance. There is a lot of work involved in acceptance.

FIVE

The Spiritual Challenge

Our Belief in the Dance

Why Me?

Standing in prayer I asked, "Why me?"
I lose, I suffer.
I lose again, I am tortured.
Repeatedly.

Why not someone else?
Why now? Why this way?

The months, the seconds are eternal,
With soft, lonely rains
Or cruel tempests.

When did this happen?
When was I abandoned?
When will I resurrect?

Children need to be hidden from me,
Friends think of leprosy,
Sisters and brothers cry in their silences,
Lovers consider infidelity.

Why me?
Through a deafening silence:
"Why not?"

Within the ongoing and challenging dimensions of living with chronic illness, we observe the physical and we feel the emotional. However, we fear and we fight the spiritual. This part of ourselves, often buried, disputed, rejected or undiscovered, contains the energy to complete the dance marathon. Perhaps because of the misuse of its "synonymous" term, religion, most challenged individuals deal with spirituality as a last resort, once all of the other business of daily living has been taken care of. We do not know how to reach our spiritual dimension, we doubt if we even have the potential to reach it, we are called *strange* by some who scoff at the spirituality of life.

Spirituality is the meaning of life. Through spirituality we attain the core of our being; we create momentum for living. An inscription on Carl Jung's front door in Switzerland reads: *Vocatus atque non vocatus deus aderit.* (Invoked or not invoked, the god is present.) Jung, considered one of the world's fathers of psychology, blended the scientific and the spiritual. If we interpret god as spirituality, that is, a sense of god without the trapping of a specific religion, then Jung believed that spirituality dwells within all of us, whether we tap into it or not. We need to integrate our spirituality with our emotionality and our physicality. A tripod balances on all three legs.

If we are to remain sane amidst the challenges of life, we need to stop regularly. Taking part in a recess allows for new energy. Unfortunately, we never stop long enough to tap into our inner life, our spiritual momentum. Productivity on the job, child rearing, being a partner, keeping ties with family, all of these "doing" things rob us of our energy. Discovering and developing our spirituality takes energy and conscious effort, time and vigor. Developing and maintaining spirituality requires a lot of work. Chronic illness can physically stop us dead in our tracks. Ironically, these limitations provide time for conscious devotion to the spiritual development essential to a fulfilled life. Whether the challenged person will grasp the opportunity depends on their motivation and their earnest desire to find their spiritual self.

Ten years of living with multiple sclerosis has convinced me that the potential for *becoming more* dwells within every chronic illness. It is a life experience which robs us of many of the choices in the "doing" department and leaves us with much potential opportunity for reflection on "being" in harmony with our life. Developing spirituality focuses on *being* as opposed to *doing*. In the silence of our soul, in the depths of our being lies our spiritual life. Chronic illness does not necessarily destroy our spirit; our spirit can flourish, given time and energy that chronic challenge brings. When illness gifts us by taking away many of the "doing" tasks, we are made available for the development of our spiritual self. All of the trivial interruptions of the material world give way to the meaningful life of our spirit.

My father sat in his chair for 27 years, paralyzed by multiple sclerosis. He was considered a wise man. He attributed his wisdom to the very fact that he sat a lot, and thought a great deal. Often, his pearls of wisdom, so simple, so straightforward, were the gift of time spent in thought. When I ventured to switch from classic studies to commerce, his calm response was, "Is this what you really want, or are you settling for the easier course?" I continued in classical studies even though it meant more years of school, because he was right; the studies led to what I really wanted. We often look to the complicated, the sophisticated, the mentally cluttered as if they possessed a magical meaning. Out of simplicity comes the complex depth of the true meaning of life, spirituality.

How ironic, how sad that for most of us it takes chronic illness or impending death to bring about spiritual energy; wellness of body and mind sometimes get in our way. Often, our spirituality evolves as we regret all the time and energy wasted on "doing" in our productive years. With the loss of bodily functions, with physical limitations, we lose control over the physical dimension of our lives. We become free to be more intent on our spirit, on our soul and the life force which springs forth from it. When nothing else makes sense to us, after all the tangible has been touched, and the logical has been thought out, we at last begin the incredible journey into the spiritual realm. When looking in books for answers, listening to television talk shows, and dialoguing with experts fail, only then do we make silence around us and listen to our inner spirituality. Thus, *the gift of illness is the potential for spiritual development.*

Our spiritual life dwells in our inner sanctum, in the silence around us. Religious devotion often invites active participation; we recite, we read, we speak. Spirituality differs in that its essence is not communicated, heard with our ears or spoken with our mouths. It just is. And when we become attuned to our soul, we become solid in our conviction of our own spirituality. Humans have built religions on tradition, on scripture, on history. That may all be very well and good, however, the spirituality I am referring to is far deeper and greater than organized religion. People acquire religion, learn religion; they experience spirituality as it lives within themselves. Religion is built by people with a particular god concept, while spirituality encompasses the core of person. Unlike religion, spirituality entails no wars, no membership, no specific practice to belong. A person's spirituality is a person's *raison d'être.*

Spirituality encompasses the meaning of life, including all of the possible god concepts. At first, the religious dogma that we have been born and programmed into has to work its way through the filtering system. This weighs on us like a tedious task, characterized by guilt and fear. Unfortunately, many religions do not separate religiosity and spirituality; too often, dogma and tradition supersede the development of spirituality. The person challenged with chronic illness must first sort out their religious experience in the light of the spirituality they seek. There is no necessity to abandon the religion that has been their tango partner for many years. Rather, there is an invitation to dance solo for a while. Progressively our spirituality will lead us into a world of concerted devotion and self-actualization; that is, grounded, focused, and more in tune with our inner spiritual life.

God Has Abandoned Me

from Sarah's diary

When my friend John showed up wearing his "roman" collar, I let him have it. "You're welcomed as a friend but not as a priest." It's fortunate that he is really a friend and understands how angry I am at this disease. He was not coming over to talk about God. Safer for him, because I think I would have thrown him out. The whole thing is rotten! How could God who supposedly loves each of us equally let this happen to me? Where is God now that I hurt so much? I told John exactly how angry I am with his God. He didn't even have an answer for me. Of course not, there is no way to forgive God for doing this to me. John just sat there and let me vent my anger. I felt better after I got all the tears, the screaming, the vile words out. He asked me if I wanted communion some time, that he would bring it over since I can't get out to church these days. I said, "Don't bother. The last thing I want is to hear, "Yes, Jesus loves me' and to pray."

Sarah experiences the typical anger and rejection that most chronic sufferers experience at the onset of their illness. People like her, who practiced their religion when able-bodied, will blame God for their illness. *When Bad Things Happen to Good People* by Harold Kushner, touches on the issues: How can a loving God allow chronic suffering, illness and death? How can God be the one to call the shots in terms of who gets chronic challenge and who does not? My understanding of our place in the universe convinces me that God has nothing to do with creating or assigning chronic illness.

We search for a target for our anger. Although God is not the appropriate target, God often gets the brunt of this anger. Chronic illnesses stem from environmental, geographical and genetic factors that together produce the conditions which affect the human body. God as the author of human life, is also the author of our freedom to choose to co-create our world. Multiple sclerosis, asthma and cancer – to name only a few – stem directly from the environment developed by humanity. Even as creator of the universe, it is not God's signature on the smog in large cities or on sexually transmitted diseases; we create our own chaos.

Through the grieving and through the anger stage, our spiritual life emerges. We hope that we have developed a relationship with a God of our own understanding, finding consolation, solace and direction in the process. Faith renders hope in tomorrow. Faith allows us to see ourselves as God-like creatures who can find the strength to learn to dance in perfect harmony with the world of our soul. We can identify with those in the scriptures who suffered, whether it be Job and his lament, or Lazarus' friends pleading to Jesus, or Jesus himself agonizing and pleading to God. We discover solidarity with fellow sufferers in the scriptures or simply come to realize that suffering and being human go hand in hand.

As part of Sarah's healing process she might consider discerning her spirituality from her religious life. She can discover answers through introspection into her strengths, her vulnerabilities and her own spiritual being: her soul. This new choreography leads to the selection of what is important in her life, to the paving of a charted way up the mountain, to the peak of a rejuvenated life. In Judaism, we learn of a handful of Israelites who dwelled on the mountain called Masada. For over one year, they held strong against their enemies until finally dying together in the name of their freedom. Climbing to the mountain to connect with a god concept is ancient. Sarah will discover and walk her own Masada, where she will be be in harmony with her spiritual strength and freedom.

How Can I Be More?

from Leah's diary

It was comforting to get a visit from Mary yesterday; this friend has not left me behind. I really need to connect with old friends since I have lost so much. At least when I get a visit, I feel normal. She brought me a book to read; actually it has nothing to do with chronic illness but everything to do with my inner life. She left a card with a note.

"When something occurs beyond chance to lead us forward in our lives, then we become more actualized people. We feel as though we are attaining what destiny is leading us to become." (The Celestine Prophecy, *p.120*)

At first I felt insulted that she suggest that I am more of a woman now than I was before I was ill; I do wish it were true. Maybe this book will teach me about spirituality, how to become spiritual.

Mary encourages Leah to read, to reflect, and hopefully to become more self-actualized. Once Leah unclutters her life of the physical limitations, the emotional roller coaster that she has been on, she can begin to find resources within herself. She will now enter the accepting stage of her illness. She has experienced the grieving stages and can now begin the process of reconstructing her life. Leah's motivation to read the material begins her inner journey.

In our self-actualization, we discover our individuality, our uniqueness, what we have to offer the world in our own signature. How do we define ourselves? Who are we?

How do we perceive our after-earth life? How do we re-energize our hope when it fades? How can we be in communion with other people?

We are potential creators of our emotional energy since it is our spiritual dimension that makes us our own unique person, with a thumb print unlike anyone else's. Visualize the following scene: it's dinner time and you check the cupboards to see what foods are there. Pasta noodles, tomato soup, mozzarella cheese. Your creativity takes over. In 15 minutes, you have a tomato-cheese pasta dish, healthy and delicious. Once the chronically challenged person checks the cupboard, way at the back where they usually do not look, they will be amazed to discover strength, intelligence, creativity and endurance they had forgotten; all are available to the challenged person.

For Leah, and for all persons ready to begin self-actualization, the imperative factor is trust: trust in ourselves to discover our spiritual potential. Most often, it will take considerable time for chronically ill persons to trust in anything or anyone, since they have been abused by the illness. Time, in its miraculous way, will usually heal our wounds so that we can begin to self-discover, with trust and hope.

Letting Go
from Bob's diary

I was talking to Marcia about how I hold on to experiences and people, hold on so tight for fear that I will lose something or someone. She said, "Join the club." Close to 40 years of my life were lived in the "grip and don't let go" mode. I like to be in control and in charge. I realize it now more than ever. I was so afraid of losing everything.

Today, I have much less control over my own life but it is funny how I feel free at the same time. I try to let go of controlling other people's lives. What an amazing feeling. When a call comes, and somebody loses it at the other end, I can hang up and say, "that has nothing to do with me."

I am vulnerable and afraid lots of times. The great thing I've found is that nobody takes advantage of me when I let them know that I am afraid or panicking. I can trust. It feels really good to let go of a lot of stuff.

Last night, I got a call from George. He is in the psychiatric hospital because he attempted suicide. His depression and the insurance company hassling him were just too much. I was scared shitless because I have to take antidepressants and I have no guarantees that my disability insurance will keep coming in every month. When my wife asked, "What's wrong, you look so pale?" I got up the courage to say, "I'm really afraid...just hold me, okay?" She did just that, held me tight and accepted that I cry for a while. Wow! It felt great to let go of that stuff. She didn't hurt me or laugh or anything other than love me as I was.

Bob's diary raises the issue of vulnerability and trust; he addresses the notion of "letting go." As part of the spiritual quest, we must learn to let go. This learning process resembles learning to ride a bicycle and trusting that as our feet let go of the ground, our balance and the bicycle wheels will keep us safe from falling down. When we let go of the control, the motion begins, we are moving. Whether we meditate or whether we visualize, as I will discuss further in this chapter, giving up control is essential. Bob's wife acknowledges his fear and encourages him to share his fear; Marcia respects his vulnerability as he lets go. In effect, Bob learns to let go in order to commune with his core being. Letting go of control leaves us open to accept the closed door in front of us; we trust in the passage through the hallway. The secret rests in patience and fearlessness; another door opens. Then we walk into a marvellous new space.

The known is more comfortable than the unknown. The unknown curses us with its void: we hesitate. The issue for chronically ill persons revolves around fear of not filling the void created by the losses. When we are diagnosed, we lose our sense of purpose. Prior to the disease, most of us defined our success in terms of our career pursuits. Our spiritual being lies dormant. Our days flash by, filled with work, hobbies, family involvement, community activity and so on. Life never halts long enough to give quiet time, indispensable to spirituality.

Sometimes, following a diagnosis, we question our value in the world, our worth. We hang on to the handle of the closed door, fighting desperately to re-open it, knowing full well that it is closed forever. We cannot abandon ourselves to the closure. Lack of trust in the natural process of life, the opening of another door, keeps us clinging to the closed one. This stage can last for months, even years. It is an agony, a barren limbo, an "in-between" state.

Desperation teaches us to trust. Progressively, confidence in the natural movement of life emerges, a trust in the orchestration of our existence is born. We can have only one door opened at one time. We must allow and accept one door to shut in order to experience new life on the other side of the next door. The time in between, while we stand between the closed doors, constitutes our time in the birth canal. Being born is not instantaneous nor painless. But this we can believe: *Once in the birth canal, we will be born.* Freedom flourishes from surrender.

"To Life, Doctor"
from Leah's diary

As the anesthesiologist ordered the nurse to begin the medication, I asked, "Can I hold Dr. Stein's hand?" As my surgeon took my hand, I said, "...that the Great Healer be with you Doctor...to life Doctor!" Dr. Stein held my hand firmly and I knew with a great certainty that we were connected each in our respective way and yet commonly to the Spirit of Life.

Our connection with a physician who shares a similar concept of spirituality makes for a strong team spirit. Both the patient and the doctor focus on a Source of healing energy, each from their own individual base.

As a patient, we should seek out a physician who has not only the training and the open approach to the illness that we are afflicted with, but also a sense of spirituality. Usually, by a simple conversation during a routine visit, we can get a clear sense of the doctor's view of the spiritual dimension. The doctor who is secure in their own competence will welcome any healing through the spiritual realm and not be intimidated by, nor question the sanity of, a patient who refuses to believe that traditional medicine contains the sole possibility for healing. I am not advocating abandonment of traditional medicine but promoting the addition of alternative medicine. If this alternative course is based on spirituality, not as a replacement but rather as an added benefit to traditional medicine, then the entire healing process is enhanced. For the patients with chronic illness, being understood and respected in their spirituality by the physician must be made a priority since the physician is a key player.

She Died Anyway

from Sarah's diary

When the news came that Jane had died, I was enraged. Sobbing uncontrollably, I told David how it was so unfair; Jane did all the "healing" things. She went to a specialized clinic for cancer patients where they taught her to imagine her cancer cells and her healthy cells. They had her do these types of things all day long. She equipped herself with a sophisticated stereo system so that she could listen to subliminal tapes for healing. Her attitude was so positive and so strong. Jane did everything the right way. I am angry, I am hurting . Jane lost all her hair three times, while she puked her guts out because of that shitty treatment. What's the point of spending all that energy for healing; she died anyway.

Sarah's disparaging entry is familiar to many of us. Probably each chronically ill person has known someone who fits this scenario, who fights nobly and wholeheartedly, only to die anyway. At this point, we seriously question the validity of the efforts put into healing. What accompanies the questioning is the resentment built up because of the false hopes.

We need to look further. Although the life itself has been lost, was its quality enhanced in any way by the patient's efforts to participate in her own healing journey ? Was Jane more content and fulfilled while doing all the "right" things as she battled her cancer? The answer is a definite yes. Challenged persons who take part in the course of their illness are motivated by a need to be active agents in what is happening to them. If you ask them, they will attest that they do not focus on the final outcome. In their daily living, in the regular effort to maintain a quality of life, they find their own options and solutions. Although doing so may never render a cure, the constant decision making and participation in their healing achieves the goal.

When we turn away from how *long* we live to how *well* we live, we begin to understand the depth of our participation in our illness and in our healing. Once we have become attuned to the changes in our lives brought on by illness, when we halt our *doing* and concentrate instead on *being*, then we find a sense of peace within the chaos. Again, *it is not how long we live, but how well we live* that matters.

Getting Grounded

from Bob's diary

I found myself becoming so agitated on the phone yesterday; my palms got all sweaty as if I was losing it. It was strange because the phone call was not necessarily that kind of encounter. I think my loss of focus is a result of neglecting my morning grounding the way my therapist taught me. When I regularly used his method, which was taking 30 minutes each morning to meditate...sometimes with music, sometimes with something I read...the rest of the day was not as much of a challenge. My most effective meditation was set during a fishing trip before my illness. We had written it together, then taped it. Usually, the rest of my day would reflect the wellness I felt during that meditation.

Bob describes a grounding exercise done each morning. It sets him in a well state of mind for the rest of the day. Opening ourself to our inner strength at the beginning of the day sets the stage for the hours to come. During the exercise, we visualize ourself as "well," with special attention paid to the ill parts of our body. Daily, repeated sessions, like the routine of any training program, create a sense of balance, of grounding so often lost in living with chronic illness.

Tapping into our spiritual dimension, or inner life, takes effort. Becoming spiritually centered does not occur by happenstance. Our days must be structured to include repetitious spiritual activity. Those of us who have never managed our time need to start now. Especially at the beginning when we do not yet see or experience the benefits, it is easy to neglect the routine. The daily practice of focusing, like many other new ventures in the waltz with chronic illness, creates easier access to our spiritual strength. (For further information on meditation and visualization techniques, see *Healing Times: A Personal Workbook* by Louise Giroux.)

On Becoming a Phoenix

In Egyptian mythology, the phoenix was a bird thought to be the servant of the sun god. Each morning at dawn, he bathed in the water, singing such beautiful songs that the sun god would stop his chariot to listen. The phoenix was unique; only one existed at a time. When the bird felt his death approaching he would build a nest, set it on fire, and let himself be consumed by the flames. After he had burned, a new phoenix would spring from the ashes and go forth from the pyre. He embalmed the ashes of his former self in an egg of myrrh and took it to the City of the Sun. There he would deposit the egg on the altar of the sun god. The phoenix was life immortalized, resurrection from the ashes, life after death.

A person living with chronic illness can be transformed into a phoenix.

Life as it was, dies. If we can let go of the old life, mourn it, allow it to be consumed by the ashes, then we can rebuild a new life through our spiritual self – a life different perhaps, but uniquely as rewarding. This new life is possible through the spiritual dimension of every person. The road to this life is one of connection with our spiritual side. The great teachings of many religions speak of the godlikeness of humanity. We are all part of the miraculous fabric that is woven with Divine thread. Illness provides the gift of a new dance. We seize the moment and see the world from a whole new vantage point, from a spiritual viewpoint. We have the chance to use a new perspective free from the binding beliefs we held prior. We rise from our own dead ashes to be new again, to be whole, to be spiritual.

SIX

Talking and Listening

Communicating the Dance

He said, She said

He said: "I feel so alone, can you sit awhile?"
She said: "Let me turn on the TV for you, I have to run."

He said: " Did you hear me?"
She said: "I wasn't talking was I?"

He said: "Pick up the phone, it keeps on ringing!"
She said: "Are you going nuts! It never rang!"

He said: "I'm dying."
She said: " You'll get over it, I'm sure.

Communication is a lifesaver. Isolation poisons life with chronic illness. Learning to talk and to listen effectively prepares the dance floor, assures harmonious music, and sets the perfect atmosphere for the dancers. Many renowned psychologists who invest their entire lives in the study of people will attest to our "social" dimension as the determinant of our adaptation to living. Experiencing oneself as "alone," apart from others, directly results from ineffective communication. Effective communication determines the quality of life for those who are challenged with chronic illness.

Contrary to popular belief that talking equals communicating, true communication consists of two domains: *talking and listening.* The latter is often underdeveloped or seriously neglected. Talking effectively necessitates learning and practicing skills and, in the same way, effective listening requires constant practice. Communication in its complex myriad of acquired and practiced skills takes time and effort; but the results show a better quality of life for all those concerned.

Effective communication should rate high among the priorities on our list, along with medication, accessibility and health care. If we are to live fully, we must learn how to communicate and we must devote time to practicing the proper techniques of good communication.

Effective talking involves more than simply speaking words – it involves our thoughts and feelings. It reflects the sum of our total awareness. Blurting out the first thing that comes into our head in an eruption of scattered thoughts can result in damaged communication; in hindsight, we regret what was said and how it was said. We're looking here at the famous, "Please engage head before mouth." Other people probably will forgive us but they will not forget, especially if they have been hurt by our words.

Effective listening incorporates our cognitive, thinking self, as well as our emotional self. Our mind should focus on what is heard while our feelings help us to connect with the talker. Often our mind gravitates toward busy-ness. We rehearse a response which in effect causes the talker to be misunderstood or purely neglected. Listening is all about partnership, since if I am to give you my undivided attention, you must be willing to give me yours when I need to be listened to.

Both the skills of talking and listening must be learned. If we are fortunate to have grown up with role models who communicated well, we might have begun our learning already. If we were raised in an atmosphere of conflict and heated talking with faulty listening, then we must erase that tape and record over it some new and effective techniques. We do not easily master effective communication.

Personally, even as a professional therapist and marriage counselor, I constantly need to practice my skills with my partner and with all those in my life. More than ever, as a chronically-ill person, I give communication an important status since I realize that it makes all the difference.

If we develop healthy and functional ways of talking and listening, nothing that comes up is unresolvable. Chronic illness with its theme song of "what now," each bar springing some new intrusion into our lives, warrants mastery of communication skills.

Communication helps us become aware of our own experience as well as that of our partner and of the other dancers in our life. Communication has everything to do with connectedness. Furthermore, no communication can take place without the engaged partnership of the two dancers. All of the situations and all of the techniques of good communication apply directly to all persons who live with chronic illness. To stand beside someone who has the illness is to live with the illness from another direction.

Sadly, the numbers of broken relationships involving persons who are chronically challenged surpass the numbers in the "unchallenged" population. There are many broken hearts who will tell you that the breakup would not have happened if the illness had not struck. I recommend that caregivers as well as persons with chronic challenge develop and maintain effective communication skills.

"I'm Talking Aren't I?"

from Leah's diary

When I was a kid, my mom called me chatter-box and that's still who I am. My girlfriend and I burn the telephone wires for hours; every night, I give her a blow by blow description of the action on The Young and Restless. *So how could this goof ball of a marriage counselor have the nerve to tell me that I don't know how to express myself? To make matters worse, my husband whined to her that I never listen to him. Why should I, he's not the one sitting all day in this goddamned chair while the world passes by. I'm really pissed off! According to Ms. Communication Know-it-all, I do not express my feelings but just blabber on and on, which is apparently annoying my poor hubby. The only reason I agreed to this counseling session was because he gave me an ultimatum. I have had no problem talking all my life; it's my legs and my eyes that are on the bum, not my freaking mouth. As for the listening, he shouldn't have anything that needs to be heard because his life hasn't been raped by this disease like mine has. The counselor also announced that my use of "you" all the time is accusatory! Oh, poor guy, he feels accused. Not only did I have to learn to cook, to wash, to get around from a chair, now I have to learn to talk* and *to listen.*

Leah's anger and resentment at the suggestion that she would do well to learn effective communication skills are normal reactions considering her childhood label of chatterbox and how she has been afflicted by her chronic condition. Nevertheless, the counselor's assessment of the couple's unhealthy communication pattern is accurate.

For Leah, the first task is to become willing to examine her learned style of talking and listening. How did her parents communicate? How was she defined as a communicator in her childhood, and in her previous career? Our definition of ourselves as effective or ineffective communicators mirrors a mixture of past experiences and present satisfaction or dissatisfaction.

Attitudes and beliefs about communication shape our relationship with it. Stereotypes such as "females are good communicators" and "males are bad communicators" are just that, stereotypes that can burden us and shape a distorted view of the possibilities of effective communication. Humans, whether male or female, need to learn how to self-disclose and how to listen to someone else self-disclose; this ability is not something we are naturally given.

The behaviors we display in communication speak loudly. The non-verbal actions we utilize – our body language, our facial expressions – form our general communication style. We may have fallen prey to influences from others in this area, from our family of origin and from personal experiences. When seriously attempting to learn effective communication skills, we can ask ourselves: what do I believe in the debate about who communicates better, men or women? What would my siblings say about me as a communicator? When have I experienced being thoroughly heard? What was it like for me to experience really listening to another person? How has my chronic illness influenced my communication? How has that illness affected my family's communication?

Some soul searching in these areas helps us focus on what we need to pay more attention to. If we deem it necessary to erase old tapes about our abilities as a communicator or about other beliefs we have on communication, then we do so. Chronic illness has the potential to alter our sex life, our parenting, our finances, our faith, our eating habits, and in the same way, it has potential to change the way in which we communicate.

The Message Equation

The goal of communication is: M=M (MESSAGE SENT = MESSAGE RECEIVED). Unfortunately, too often the equation goes something like: M=m or m=M or m=m. Let's look at examples of these equations.

M=m: Leah says, "Shut the blinds, I just want to die today."
Husband replies, "Boy are these blinds dusty or what."
The MESSAGE given here was important and was not the trivial message received and returned. Therefore, no effective communication took place.

m=M: Leah says, "I'll have a nap and then we can go out for coffee."
Husband replies, "Why are you always rejecting me like this!"
The message here was informal, yet the MESSAGE received was blown way out of proportion.

m=m: Leah says, "Do you want to watch a movie?"
Husband says, "Sure, as soon as I put away this stuff."
The message sent here was light and the message received here was light also. This exchange was effective.

M=M: Leah says, "Shut the blinds, I just want to die today."
Husband says, "I'm here, tell me...it must be bad right now."
This MESSAGE, even if more serious than the previous, was effectively transmitted because it was the same as the MESSAGE received. Again, this exchange was effective.

The concept of the message equation is that the message sent should equal the message received; this equality relates the significance or weight of the content. In most instances of miscommunication, the problem lies in this equality imbalance, where the message sent and the message received are not equal strength.

Messages come in different intensities. There are also different types or kinds of messages. These include topic messages that focus on things, events, ideas, places, people who are not present in the conversation. Self-messages focus on me as person, my experiences, my thoughts and my feelings, my wants and my actions. Partner-messages focus on you as a person, when I express something about you; while relationship messages communicate about my personal involvement with others. All of these types of messages can be effective in their own right. Paralleling the "sent" and the "received" message constitutes the art of communication.

One of the ineffective patterns that Leah displays is her invalidating statements toward her partner, whose self-esteem diminishes because of her negative comments. It appears that she discounts her partner's needs to be heard while she takes center stage. Also, she assumes that she has priority to be heard because of her challenge. Of course, this is totally dysfunctional. Self-other esteem attitudes have to do with the value I attribute to myself when I place myself in our partnership and the value I attribute to you when I place you in our partnership. The goal is to count myself as equally important to you and to count you as equally important to myself. Let's look at the four possible positions:

I don't count me, I don't count you
I count me, I don't count you
I don't count me, I count you
I count me, I count you.

I don't count me, I don't count you:

Leah says, "I can't handle this depression and you are just as depressed; we're sinking each other."

I count me, I don't count you:

Leah says, "Let me handle the disability people, you'll break down."

I don't count me, I count you:

Leah says, "This illness has taken away all my emotional energy; thank God you're so much stronger than me."

I count me, I count you:

Leah says, "This is rough but I know that together, if we pool our strengths, we can make it."

In effective communication, both parties value each other with genuine reciprocal esteem. They evaluate themselves positively and honor their partner in the same way.

Of course, *we are who we were*. Chronic illness does not magically turn non-effective communicators into effective ones. We tend to forget that many of the challenges stemming from communication will be found to be old ones. Too often, illness becomes the excuse. If we practice using statements that are "counting," these increase our self-esteem; we validate ourselves and affirm our partners when we apply the same kind of positive statements to them. It is guaranteed that this pattern will yield positive attitudes towards self-acceptance, the hallmark of emotional and mental health.

Talking It All Out Feels So Much Better

from Sarah' s diary

Talk about talking it out! My doctor finally took time to listen today so I finally feel greatly relieved. Nothing has changed in my physical situation, but just to be able to say how this disease affects me in all the areas of my life, has made all the difference. I confessed that I had been feeling more depressed than usual; he explained to me about changing to another antidepressant and maybe getting more sun and fresh air regularly. When he asked about my opinion on antidepressants, I said exactly what I think. "Sometimes I hurt too much in my heart...too much feeling down and out...I think antidepressants have their place in helping me cope." I could see in his face how he understood me and I think he also picked up in my eyes that I was genuine.

It was the best thing to do, to ask him, right out when I got here, if he could take time to sit with me for a few minutes. I did this, which some people might find somewhat controlling, because he always runs around as if he has a little tag on his forehead that says, "Busy, busy...get on with it." At this point in my life as an invalid, I want to strive for quality, even if that sounds weird. What I really want is to enjoy the little bits of peace and the people in my life as much as I can. I could hardly believe how thoroughly talked out I felt after that talk with my doctor. It was as if every aspect of who I am and how I am living came out. The complaints are still there, the illness sure as heck has not gone away, but somehow I feel that I can go on a little easier now.

What Sarah describes here is her experience of total self-disclosure and heightened self-awareness. Without realizing the mechanics involved, which five elements of the self make up a total disclosure, Sarah intuitively assessed her personal and total awareness and disclosed her thoughts, her feelings, her actions, her wants, and her senses. All she knows is that she feels better as a result of having done that. We can compare the result to the experience of satiety after a gastronomically delightful meal, with all the fixings, our favorite drink, and dessert. The complete disclosure of our experience can be compared to the statement, "There, it is finished."

Identifying what is going on internally and communicating that awareness engages our thoughts, our feelings, our actions, our desires and our senses on any given issue. We communicate these five components in any order in which they make their way into our conscious awareness. Consequently, we talk each element out, mention each one as we aim at full self-disclosure. This entire disclosure will relieve us as well as be a valuable insight for our listener. Because of our pattern of talk, which has been influenced and formed from past experiences, we usually find ourselves automatically selective when we self-disclose. Some people talk feelings more than thoughts, or avoid expressing wants, thinking that their desires are unjustified. Here, the quality of the relationship with our listener often determines how thorough we can actually be. We always wonder about how our messages will be received and communicate accordingly. In the best of circumstances, we experience safety and security in totally self-disclosing without fear of rejection or retribution. We will do well to remember that we are "talking," that no action must take place after the dialogue. We need, and justifiably so, to express our total experience.

When we undertake total self-disclosure, we involve all five elements of our awareness; we make five short statements, one for each element, as our listener simply *listens.* No crosstalk or gestures from the listener interrupt our self-disclosure. After we have communicated our message, the listener can appropriately send back our message and subsequently share with us what they are experiencing. In many situations, we can gain as much relief by writing down our self-awareness messages. The results are the same; we have expressed ourselves more thoroughly.

I think: this is a thought statement.

Sarah, "I think antidepressants have their place..."

Thinking denotes a mental activity that occurs continuously, even when we dream. Our thoughts are the mental conversations we have with ourselves. Usually, most people have no difficulty in expressing their thoughts, given a safe environment where they do not fear how their thoughts will be received. Usually thoughts imply scripts embedded in our minds; even though they may be negative, we cannot deny their presence. The only way we can eradicate an unwanted thought is by saying it out, and then replacing it with other types of more positive thoughts. This kind of self-talk with our thoughts can improve our inner life.

I feel: this is a feeling statement.

Sarah, " I had been feeling more depressed..."

The absolutely most important feature of this element is that *a feeling is not good, not bad, it just is.* We may have been socialized as children to ward off so-called negative feelings, or influenced not to express them. In reality, our feeling self equates with our emotional life, an inward automated system that exists totally apart from our thinking processes. We may think that we "should" be grateful for food on our table, but our feeling of abandonment because the kids are all gone at dinner takes the leading role.

The only effective way to deal with a feeling lies in the acknowledgement of it and in talking it out. It loses its impetus and its strength once it is revealed. Chronically ill persons often experience overwhelming sad feelings, frightening feelings and other types of emotions that are difficult to deal with. This condition can derive from the medical challenge itself or from the medication. The chemical products to relieve symptoms, to cure an illness or to halt the progression of disease, play havoc on the emotional stability of the person. Nevertheless, the only way to tame the feelings, whatever they may be, is to talk them out, without fear. Doing this conjures up images of deflating a balloon. Little by little, as we release the pent-up feelings, the problem shrivels.

I do, I did: this is an action statement.

Sarah, "...to ask him right out, if he had time..."

Recognizing what we have done already concerning an issue and deciding what move we would like to do empowers us. Taking action dignifies us and transfers us from a sitting position, in a wheelchair for example, to a more proactive position on our mental feet. Some caregivers rob their patients of the power to make choices. Even the minutest of decisions, whether to wear a green gown or a blue one, whether to have mozzarella cheese or cheddar cheese, whether to watch this program or that program, creates a sense of individual power that a chronically ill sufferer desperately needs.

I want: this is a desire statement.

Sarah, "I want quality in my life..."

Sometimes, when we express ourselves, we fear our wants, thinking that we will be construed as spoiled or complaining. Our wants are probably legitimate and in reality just because we disclose them, we do not usually expect the other to meet them. What we like, what we want, what we intend, what we wish, what we don't want often lie hidden because they are considered umimportant.

But our wants help generate options for choices and for organizing ourselves. It is a case of being honest with ourselves. Actions stem from desires; what we are doing, preparing to do, or have done helps us understand what we want and vice versa. Our intentions genuinely indicate where to go from here.

I see, I hear, I touch, I smell, I taste: these are sense statements.

Sarah, "I could see in his face that he understood..."

Our senses connect us to the outside world and they never lie. Most often, from seeing or hearing, we gain the first form of a message coming in. When chronic illness hits, our senses can be altered. At times, certain medications will affect our hearing; we will hear ringing that isn't there. We may have a heightened sense of taste or develop an intolerance for noise, as in the case of many who suffer neurological illnesses. If we can effectively communicate these sense-statements, we have already diminished their impact on us. On the positive side, using our senses to create a healing environment can be wonderful. A scented candle can become a visual and an olfactory anchor and an important focus for relaxing. Soothing music provides calm and serenity when we need to tune out the kids arguing among themselves. We can escape turmoil through our senses. This form of communication with self takes on the face of a communion with our inner world.

Total self-awareness and self-disclosure heals us. In the world of health care, it provides the best tool for self-care. We want to remain in charge of our lives even though often, our chronic illness fights for the lead. We can *take the lead.* If we can use the five dimensions – the want, the action, the feeling, the thought, the sensing – and disclose what we are experiencing at any given time, we will connect with ourselves as our own best caregiver. People around us will benefit greatly from a less confused patient and hopefully will join us in their own self-disclosure.

U-Turn Talk Gets Us Nowhere!
from Bob's diary

If I make small talk, she says I never tell her about my feelings. The truth is, I was never one to open up much, not before I got sick and sure not now. When my wife comes home from work, I talk her ears off because I'm alone all day. She says it's annoying because I go on and on about unimportant stuff. Last night, we got into a really heavy argument; she was totally angry and kept accusing me with "You do this...you don't do that...you are feeling sorry for yourself..."

You better believe that I wasn't going to take it lying down. I told her what I thought of her, "You don't know the first thing about being alone all the time...you are so caught up in your freaking job...You always put on a mean face when I ask you to bring me something..."

The whole night was one big fight with us going back and forth until I got so exhausted and went to bed. This morning, we both pretended that nothing happened, and went to the small stuff again. This sucks! I don't know how to get through to her anymore and she probably feels the same way.

One of the most poisonous hindrances to effective communication is the U-TURN message. In its place people should use I-FOCUS statements. To speak for myself means owning up to what I send and taking responsibility for the content of my message. As a result, messages are clearer and easier for my listener to hear. If Bob had said, "I feel deeply alone all day," an I-FOCUS statement, instead of saying, "You don t know anything about loneliness," a U-TURN statement, his message would have been received quite differently. People are much more apt to accept a message delivered from the "I" position. This does not mean that when I speak for myself I focus solely on me; I can express my own awareness on a topic, on another person or on a relationship. The prime determiner of the quality and effectiveness of my statements lies in my positive regard and positive intention.

Both Bob and his wife have fallen prey to U-TURN statements that provoke defensiveness in the listener. What starts out with a YOU, usually comes right back at me, hitting me in the face. The other person, who experiences feeling attacked or boxed in, resists. Who likes their life to be run by another? The U-TURN statement results in a "right back at you" message. Most people find these types of messages invasive, pushy or manipulative; little wonder, this style works against effective communication. The listener finds it necessary to recoil, to defend and to protect themself. It is a vicious circle.

We all talk in one of four styles, among which we drift in and out, depending on the circumstances of the message and the content of that message.

Are you a "surface" talker? Do you dance around an issue?
Are you a "my way or the highway" talker? The French throw-around dance.
Are you an "explorer" talker? Beautiful sweeping ballroom dance.
Are you a "straight-shooter" talker? Fred Astaire and Ginger Rogers.

The first style, the *surface* talker rattles on and on or simply uses very short informative messages. Often, this is a person who prefers to not talk about feelings. Reporting on how the nurse's visit went, describing the physio exercise, making a joke about the doctor's new assistant, telling the story of how the wheelchair got caught in the snow, visiting with a neighbor are all examples of this style of small talk. Making proper use of this basic style of talking can be perfectly appropriate depending on what is needed. If a chronically ill person communicates solely in this basic style, there may be genuine concern from the caregiver as to the degree the patient is expressing their emotional health. This is the complaint that Bob's wife gives, that he never talks about his feelings, but rather stays safely in surface talk.

"It's my way or the highway." Sadly enough, too many of us have received messages which aim at controlling. One famous line from family members is, "I know exactly what pills you should take." Giving advice, teaching, or selling constitute forms of this forceful style. Sometimes the message is propelled actively and at other times it is indirectly sent. If Bob's wife withholds sexual attention because he attacked her verbally, she sends the "my way or the highway" type of message. If on the other hand, his wife complains incessantly about what he does or does not do, criticizes him for his annoying small talk or disqualifies him as able to make decisions about his yoga classes for relaxation, she uses direct controlling talk. The more blatant ways to communicate with forcefulness are by using blaming, demanding, accusing, threatening and labeling statements. Once aware of the potential damages that this talking style delivers, Bob and his wife probably would be wise to abandon it, since it appears that their pet style has led to their communication breakdown.

One of the much more profitable talking styles is the *"explorer"* type. While using it, people search for possible avenues to follow. Giving impressions of an issue, explaining how such or such an issue affects each person, or brainstorming together can generate solid and effective results. If Bob used statements like, "I know that I don't talk about my feelings much and wonder why they scare me so much," or "Have you ever experienced loneliness?" or "I detect from your face some frustration when I ask you to bring me something; am I right?" the outcome would undoubtedly become fruitful. This style would lend itself wonderfully to the two sitting together for a brainstorming session on how they could possibly relieve the tension and work on their communication rather than sweeping the problem under the carpet.

The *"straight-shooter"* talker is direct, uses I-FOCUS statements, and usually attracts favorable responses from their listener. This style of talking lends itself more to important discussion of issues. It incorporates observations given in a sharing atmosphere: each listens to the other and accepts them at face value. It is the ideal situation.

Somehow, if Bob and his partner could be motivated to take the necessary time and necessary emotional energy to undertake straight-shooting talk, the bridge would form between them and prevent them from falling into the moat that presently drowns them. Most likely, neither one of them has practiced this type of compassionate talking; the skills would take time to learn as well as to practice. I would recommend a coach in this circumstance, someone qualified to help them learn the specifics of effective communication.

It's not what *we say that causes havoc, it's* how *we say it.* Any message, any content can be effectively communicated. There is nothing too horrifying, too crude, too private that cannot be disclosed if appropriate styles of talking are used. For a chronically ill person, the first order of business might very well be to explore which pattern of talk constitutes our general conversations. From there, if we are committed to communication, we can alter, add, take away or customize an effective style. Talking effectively takes on more importance when we are ill; our caregiver, our family, our doctor, our nurse, our minister, our friends, all those with whom we need to share our experience will come through for us if we become master talkers.

The Art of Listening

from Leah's diary

I haven't slept for three nights. I feel like crawling out of my skin because of the steroid the Doc prescribed for my attack. Because my husband has been down this road before, he refuses to take time to listen to my complaints; as far as he is con-

cerned, I sound like a broken record. He never sits long enough to hear me out. If I tie him down, his eyes are everywhere but on me. It's so rough for me to start to talk, I wish he could draw me out more; sometimes, being sought out would make me feel cared for instead of neglected.

This morning, he sort of listened while he sipped his coffee but then when he answered me, the stuff coming out was not what I had said; he did not understand. He asked me, "Do you want your toast now or later, to take with your prednisone?" I didn't even want toast! Why couldn't he ask me what I wanted to eat; I was more in the mood for cereal. Maybe I am going crazy like he says. Actually, no. He doesn't listen to me, I am not heard and I am totally alone.

In this sad journal entry, Leah's keen awareness of a listening problem between her and her caregiver generates sorrow. Her husband is most likely naive about which patterns of listening are ineffective and how he could learn more effective listening skills. Leah would gain much by learning the mastery of listening herself so that both of them could dance harmoniously together in the hearing part of their communication. When we effectively listen, we use five different skills:

I am beside you: let's dance cheek to cheek.
I recognize you: our bodies step together.
I ask you to disclose: the twirl.
I summarize your message: the grand finale.
I question you: would you care to dance again?

I am beside you...

When Leah reports that her husband cannot keep eye contact when he listens, she refers to the initial stage of listening. Listening entails active involvement. In order to achieve this, we need for the moment to suspend our needs, to give the other our undivided attention. It may be difficult to get used to since we are better trained in rehearsing responses than in just taking it all in.

We can show that we are listening by our body language, by looking directly at the person, by nodding our head, by showing that we are indeed intent on listening to their experience. We listen also by touching the other at times; we use moments of physical closeness to try to tune in to the other. It appears that Leah's partner lacks motivation in the listening area, that if he were willing to take the time, she would experience him as truly listening to her.

I recognize you...

Recognizing someone you meet means conveying the message to them that they have been noticed. While Leah attempts to tell her husband about the awful side effects of the prednisone, something from him like "That sounds awful," or "I can see you're going through a rough time," or "No kidding, that stuff sounds poisonous," would have signaled that she was indeed being heard. When we tune in to our partner's energy and the emotional content of what they say, we send back, briefly, some kind of acknowledgement. We focus on the talker, we get in touch with where they are coming from, and from which zone of their experience they are talking. We call it empathy, the cornerstone of all listening to another, whether to a sick child, a patient, a client, a spouse or a friend. Empathy gifts the person with acceptance, understanding and affirmation.

Leah's husband probably blocks his listening because he feels unable to take the emotional charge that this listening would produce. To stay beside someone, not in front of, not behind, but beside, while they talk of their painful experience, takes courage. We experience helplessness. However, not running away but remaining beside them is the richest form of compassion and respect of the other's dignity.

I ask you to disclose...

If Leah and her partner could take time and energy for attentive listening, they could move forward to the questioning stage. Her frustration stems from the questions posed in a closed style, for example when he says, "Do you want your toast now or later?" She becomes frustrated because she has not been given the option of choosing which food she wants. Her husband used a closed question, the type that warrants only a "yes" or "no" response. It is closed because he assumes she will have toast and doesn't allow her to express an alternative. Rephrasing the question as, "What would you like to eat this morning?" would have given Leah the dignity of choice.

As chronically ill persons, we need to have a say in as many things as possible, given the controls and limits the illness forces on us. When we ask someone to disclose more, we invite them to continue talking and simultaneously we confirm that we are beside them for as long as they need to talk.

Some very basic yet extremely effective questions that Leah's caregiver could ask are "Tell me what you think about when you can't sleep at night? or "What went on in your mind when the Doc first told you he was putting you on prednisone?" or "How can I help you?" By the vehicle of these open-ended questions, Leah would experience messages of genuine caring, and of genuine interest about what she is going through.

I summarize your message...

When her husband sent back her message, Leah found it distorted. This is an extremely disappointing situation for the talker. If a listener says, "Let me see if I understand...," then the talker can check the response and add, "Well, not exactly, here's what I said/meant..." In order to ensure that I have understood your message, I summarize as often as possible during our conversation without making it a hindrance to the self-disclosure. Ensuring of the accuracy of the content – *message sent = message received* – protects effectiveness. Maybe Leah's husband does not think that she sounds like a broken record; maybe she would do well to check things out with him. At this stage of effective listening, we repeat, by using the other's words or by paraphrasing, what we have heard to confirm and clarify the message.

I question you...

By the looks of things, Leah would welcome an interested question or two about how this experience unfolds for her. Open questions such as those discussed in "I ask you to disclose" are the best. The listener attempts to gather or fill missing information at this point.

The "why" question should be avoided since it creates a defensiveness, a "Why not!" type of answer. These questions can feel like a challenge because they call on the talker to justify what they have said. Better forms of questioning use "How" because it leaves the air free of all constraints.

For Leah and her spouse, an agreed-upon time to talk with each other would probably be more effective, since they have different living styles and time constraints. After some sharing and effective listening, both would feel more encouraged to share deeper feelings because they feel good about each other. Leah and her dance partner would win first place at the dance marathon, having learned and practiced the steps to effective communication. If they learn to listen, they will hear each other; they will communicate.

Arguing Fair
from Bob's diary

If this keeps up between the kids, me and their mother, I'm asking the Doc to put me in the hospital. The shooting match was so terrible that my breath stopped. I was wheezing, trying to catch it; not to mention feeling pain in my chest and sweating like a pig. My wife always brings up every single thing I failed to do for the kids when I was well. "This is why they don't respect you now, you didn't earn their respect before you were sick."

The whole thing started when I asked Billy to go out to get me a newspaper. Mr. Important did not have time for that, what with talking for hours on the phone with his girlfriend. The first thing I knew, my wife was yelling and screaming about when he was a baby! I tried to counterattack, even though I was shaking, but that made matters worse. At one point, I thought my wife had lost it when she picked up the ladle and motioned as if she would throw it at Billy or at me; it was scary to see her eyes bulging out of her head.

This problem is old, about me and the kids and how I have problems with them. When I was a kid, my dad never argued with my mom, and whenever she would begin to get down on him, he would leave. One of my uncles was so violent, that whenever he drank he would fist fight with somebody. Once, I hid in a closet while he and my dad went at it.

Something has to be done. There must be a way that we could try to resolve this because I need peace for my attacks to subside.

Conflict is natural and to be expected in any type of relationship. We must learn to deal with it appropriately because in its inevitability, it will take up residence in our lives with chronic illness. An interesting approach to begin with lies in delving into our reaction patterns, how do we usually behave when someone disagrees with us about something. What happens when we think of negotiating an issue? The most important outcome of resolving conflict is that it summons up maturity so that no one wins or loses in the situation, but rather both parties come to an acceptable difference. Unfortunately, too often, we have a goal in mind: to win. The need to win colors and poisons any productive dialogue and effective listening. Arguing is an acquired skill, not inherent to us, but rather a technique we learn, develop and practice throughout our lives. Chronic illness will stir feelings, problematic situations and old hurts like nothing else ever has. A heap of homework sends us to the drawing board to learn how to argue.

What Bob relates in his diary entry is a classic situation for the family system living with the challenge of chronic illness; everyone suffers. Clearly, neither Bob nor his spouse nor his son know effective ways to deal with "hot" issues.

Rule no.1 ***Keep to the here and now.*** **Keep in step with the music.**

When Bob's wife brings up the history of his parenting, she breaks the rule of "*here*" and "*now.*" Using yesterday's problems as today's ammunition usually compounds the issue by implicitly bringing up past failures. Often, people sit on past grudges or resentments and give in to their impulses to discharge their venom. The past has no place in arguing fairly. If she feels a great need to address the issue of Bob's parenting, his wife would gain more by setting time and energy aside for a straight heart-to-heart talk with him, a straight-shooter conversation nowhere near the heated argument stage of their communication.

Rule no. 2 ***Keep to one issue.*** **Cha-cha or waltz.**

As we imagine the scene in Bob's home, we see zingers shooting every which way and a barrage of topics being thrown around helter-skelter. If the couple had been somehow able to identify and discuss calmly one specific issue, say Billy's unavailability to help out, this issue would be the focus of the conflict-resolution session. Bob's bad record as a parent would not even enter into the picture. Bob's experience would be redefined, without need to defend himself or to attack his wife in a countersuit. Keeping to one issue creates safety and a secure atmosphere for all who are concerned in the argument.

Rule no. 3 *Use "I," forget about "counterattack."* Lead me into dance, don't shove me.

The same characteristics of I-focus messages that were mentioned previously apply in the case of fighting fair. We stick to our personal responsibility concerning the issue, without resorting to the U-turn technique, which inevitably boomerangs. Attacks on our partner, about their behavior or their temperament, produce war zones. In a fair argument if Bob's wife communicates a genuine complaint using an "I" statement such as, "I notice the friction between you and Billy, can I help?" he would listen without need to counterattack her. We can usually accept reproof graciously when it is due. Sometimes, the game of mind reading plays havoc on our conflict resolution. Checking things out solves the problem of wondering what exactly our partner has in mind to discuss.

Rule no. 4 *Keep emotions appropriate.* You're wearing cowboy boots to tango?

What a frightening situation to imagine the ladle flying around in the kitchen in the midst of the verbal confrontation and psychological violence! Emotions explode readily when conflict erupts. Feelings that have been pent up for a long time take over and people say and do irrational things, even abusive and dangerous things. Gauging our feelings must precede any attempt at resolving conflict. Extremely helpful as it may be to express feelings while fighting fair, the feelings must be confined to an appropriate size for the issue. Unrestrained, uncontrolled venting leads to violence, whether that violence be verbal, psychological, or physical. Obviously, Bob's wife has been harboring strong emotions; she needs catharsis, but not in this particular instant. Choosing another avenue for herself to vent, to calm down and to communicate what is pent up would be a perfectly acceptable future endeavor.

Rule no. 5 *Don't try to win.* Dance to the same rhythm.

When one person wins, another loses; and when one loses, both lose. The goal in resolving differences is to find a mutually satisfactory solution to the problem at hand, so that all parties come out as winners. In this particular situation, Bob's request for a newspaper constitutes an acceptable want. Billy's refusal to take time to cooperate is unacceptable, and just as inappropriate is mom's tirade over the past and her use of a ladle. If mom and dad could talk calmly to Billy, explaining that they need his help, it would be a great start. Next, Bob and his spouse could go on to resolving the parenting issue that undermines this outburst. Maybe Billy will remain uncooperative. However, Bob could find another way of getting his newspaper without losing the conflict; mom would win since she could process her experience.

Given an ideal situation where Bob and his wife would effectively attempt to resolve the conflict, the dance might go something like this:

- they would clearly identify what the issue is
- they would set up a contract together, when, where and what they would discuss
- they would assure a clear understanding of each other's position
- they would identify what they want
- they would generate a list of possible actions to take
- they would choose one item from the list generated
- they would test out their plan
- they would evaluate the outcome.

What is making Bob ill is not that conflict exists in his household, but rather that no one knows how to handle the conflict. The multitude of intrusions stemming from a home where chronic illness has taken residence have potential to destroy the lives of the persons sharing that home. Acquiring conflict resolution skills makes the difference between making it, or breaking under it.

Talking without Speaking
from Sarah's diary

When I found my son's note on my desk, "World's Greatest Mom," my heart pounded. That kid of mine doesn't talk much, but he sure says a lot. I guess all the hugs I've been sneaking by him have paid off. Lately, when I feel a need for affection, I am bolder than before and just reach out and hug him or his father. It was weird last night that, just as I was feeling teary, my husband picked up on it; he came and sat with me, put his arm around me. Let me tell you, that was worth far more than a long speech of what he felt. I knew it without needing to hear a word. More and more, I am getting in tune with my own signals too; my body talks to me and I hear it when I listen. When I began spring cleaning last week, my head started to spin and sure enough, it was time to take a break. After my nap that day, a florist delivered flowers from my good friend who had heard that I was under the weather. What a wonderful feeling to be so nurtured; it makes me feel healthy.

Sarah and her family share nonverbal communication; they effectively tune in to one another. They are fortunate, but they work for it from what we read here. When life unfolds within the realm of chronic illness, it drags us into muddy waters, dark tunnels, and bottomless pits; in these times, nonverbal talking can be most effective. With our eyes we connect with the inner world of another, with our arms we comfort each other, with our actions we reach out and connect even though we are not physically there. Words limit talking. Body language in its unlimited variations never lets us down.

What sounds particularly interesting about Sarah's entry is her symbiosis with her own body. Obviously she has learned to recognize the signals, the bells and whistles that her body sounds when it wants to get her attention. Disease constantly stimulates the body in some fashion or another; medication does the same thing. A chronically ill person under constant bombardment from both the illness and from the attempts at cure or relief of symptoms picks up all sorts of physical cues. Taking deep breaths, focusing the mind, relaxing the muscles, all set the stage for body communication. If we listen, we will hear, so loudly at times, that our body will deafen our silence. Contrary to the assumption that our body is less-than because it is diseased, we discover that our body is better equipped than ever to communicate. Too often, we abandon it. It does not abandon us.

The poem "He said, She said" that introduces this chapter on communication concludes on a gruesome note of suicidal proportion. We gather that he experiences suicidal thoughts and that she remains oblivious to the severity of his message. Both he and she communicate ineffectively.

The possibility of taking one's own life, when living with chronic illness, plagues us. Sometimes we experience exhaustion from struggling to walk, struggling to sleep, struggling to get medical attention, struggling with our broken heart. It is then, under the abominable pressure of the struggle, that we can fall prey to the desire to bail out. Without effective communication, both from the person with the illness and from those who share their life, doom takes over.

The best preventive medicine for desperation is talking and listening clearly. Realizing how serious the issue of communication actually is, we must motivate ourselves to explore the skills and summon the courage to end our isolation. Although illness takes us as hostages in the deep woods of despair, we still maintain our inherent drive to be connected with ourselves and with each other. The journey takes on the allure of a hand-in-hand walk through a sunfilled clearing of hopeful connectedness.

SEVEN

Holistic Wellness

Dancing with Chronic Illness

Holistic Wellness

No sound, void of music,
Speaker wires crossed, not connected.
No song, no harmony,
Wrong side of CD on track.
Still nothing heard,
The dog pulled the plug from the wall.

I cannot hear the music.
I cannot dance.

No energy, legs are weak,
No one to walk toward.
Hopelessness ravishes the heart,
Motivation, attitude, have died.
There is no God.
The sham is over, transformed into harsh reality.

I cannot hear the music.
I cannot dance.
Taking time to sleep, to rejuvenate,
Respecting limitations, stretching wisely.
Touched by a child's spirit
Falling in love with me, for the first time.
Climbing the snake path, reaching Masada,
New Birth canal, Resurrection.

I hear music.
I am dancing.

Chronic illness does not necessarily make a person un-well. We can attain wellness not only in some areas, but wholly, when we integrate all of our three dimensions and when we practice patience with the ebb and flow of the process involved in being an active member of our wellness team.

Renewal is not static, nor is it passive; it requires a dynamic attitude toward chronic illness, born of all the past struggles with the disease. Furthermore, renewal, with its ever-changing character, demands alertness as well as increased self-awareness; it puts that self-awareness to the test. One of the hallmarks of this renewal is a person's hard-won ability to separate themselves from the illness. The first order of business of self-renewal and of actually learning to dance with chronic illness lies in understanding what the term holistic suggests. Next we need to apply this principle of wholeness to each dimension of our wellness.

The Concise Oxford Dictionary (9th edition) defines *whole* as:

an uninjured, unbroken, intact state
not less than
with no part removed
all there is of a thing
a unity, not as separated parts.

The Concise Oxford Dictionary (9th edition) defines *well* as:

in a satisfactory way
in the right way
thoroughly, extensively, favourably
in good health
with no loss of advantage.

Notice that the concept of wellness does not mean free of limitations, totally perfect. Rather, the term implies a degree of acceptability or satisfaction. Therefore, to be in a state of wellness is to be in a frame of mind and a frame of heart and soul that accepts one's physical limitations. The concept of wholeness also suggests a coherent working together of all the constituent parts of the organism. When heaviness of heart plagues someone, when the grieving of losses saddens that person, we can be certain that physical wellness suffers as well, as does spiritual and cognitive wellness. We strive to achieve an acceptable level of comfort in all three dimensions of well-being. It is then that we will dance with holistic wellness.

Physical Wellness

Although the onset of chronic illness may be preceded by emotional stress of some sort, the first manifestations of illness are usually physical. The body collapses first.

In order to take proper care of and to participate *in* our physical wellness, we need to seek appropriate medical treatment. Gone are the days of pledging allegiance to the "one and only one" family physician. Today, we can interview our physician upon onset of illness. We can ask "Are you familiar with this illness? Do you have experience with this illness? Do you accept me as a patient with this illness and all that this might entail?" An honest and open session with our family physician opens the door to a new relationship that takes into account the needs of each member of our family as well as the common goal: holistic wellness. Even though most of us who live with chronic illness have a variety of specialists – from neurologist, to urologist, opthalmologist to psychiatrist – I believe that the family physician remains the most important member of one's medical team. As we establish ownership of our lives we need to seek the best possible medical treatment and the most competent professional healthcare workers as part of our wellness team.

In the interests of our quality of life and our overall well-being, we need to seek out appropriate housing that meets our needs. When climbing the stairs at night or taking naps during the day zaps away energy that we could use for something more constructive, we owe it to ourselves to make a change. Many financial assistance programs exist which can help us in renovating our homes. If need be, we should move. When it comes to bathing, a small shower stool can help us with the possible physical challenges of carrying out our personal hygiene. When cooking while standing up becomes problematic, we can get a chair on wheels to scoot around the kitchen.

The key to physical wellness resides mainly in respect for our limitations. First, we recognize the physical losses, then we effectively grieve those losses and move on to work with what remains.

If a chronically ill person aims at achieving holistic wellness, then time and energy management take precedence over most other management skills. Depending on the natural temperament of the challenged individual, managing daily life can be more or less demanding at first. With many illnesses, physical energy is quickly consumed because most chronic illnesses make the body weak. Every morning, the wise chronically challenged person sets up the day in a way that will allow them to tap into energy when needed. If mom makes it a priority to cheer her son at the basketball court around 4:00 p.m., then she will probably need to save a lot of energy prior to that time; she may nap, restrain from walking too much, or keep her work schedule light. Planning for next week's or next month's events requires the same technique. Allowing extra days for rest when traveling shows wise management of time and energy. Because the chronically challenged person has suffered many painful losses, the important events and activities of life in the present should be prioritized. We achieve more goals with proper time and energy management. Selection of activities may be necessary and we may finally learn that challenging two-letter word: NO, which many of us do not utilize soon enough.

Constant self-care approach and sound practice of time and energy management sets the stage for a well choreographed routine.

Emotional Wellness

The female professional model knows that her base coat of make-up means everything; this basic undercoat allows her colors to be sharp, her eyes to stand out, her cheekbones to be stunning. In the emotional realm a person's base coat means *attitude.*

Without a positive attitude, chronic illness invades and conquers. A positive attitude translates as a frame of mind, a spontaneous immediate way of thinking that sees the potential, the good, the hope in anything. Skeptics may be inclined to write this off as eternal optimism. In fact, if our attitude displays itself as anything less than positive, we might as well curl up and forget about trying to live a full life. So let's distinguish between a positive attitude and a Pollyana-ish attitude. The latter bases itself on naivety and ignorance while the first is based on realistic observation, proper ownership of the situation, choices made in a reflective way and finally a decision to take the positive avenue.

For the person not naturally inclined or programmed to live or think positively here are some steps that might be taken:

- with any given situation, realistically observe the facts of the situation
- when you are weighed down by incomplete grieving then continue the process
- do some form of letting go, whether crying or anger work
- during this process, take responsibility for how this situation affects you
- look at all the options leading to a solution; perhaps the status quo presents the best solution

- decide to take a positive outlook on the awareness you've gained
- remember that good can come from any situation
- learn that good doesn't necessarily mean feel good.

Growth for human beings occurs in great spurts during painful times; we stretch our limits and become more than we have been. A positive attitude can cure or maintain stability in the progression of a disease; holistic wellness manifests itself through a positive attitude.

Chronic illness triggers depression. This hallmark of emotional challenge undermines much of the quality of life of a chronically ill person. We need to identify from which form of depression we suffer. Is our depression induced by our illness? Does our illness attack our mood center? Is our depression brought on by a culmination of stressful events?

When our mood center and the neurological chemical elements of the brain malfunction, we suffer from chemical depression. Proper medication will alleviate this form of depression. Gone are the days when a stigma was attached to taking antidepressants for chemical depression. In essence, taking insulin for diabetes and taking antidepressants for chemical depression add up to the same thing.

If certain circumstances and situations in our life are causing the depression, usually a manifestation of repressed anger, then therapy might be in order. This will allow us to let go of the anger and to reduce the situational depression. A family physician can distinguish which type of depression we suffer from and how we can go about getting treatment. Mood has everything to do with wellness; if our mood is up and positive, then emotional wellness will prevail.

As part of normal and healthy daily living, we experience anger. However, unmanaged anger, resulting in abusive behavior, does not make for healthy daily living. By "abusive" I refer to verbal, nonverbal or physical behavior that lessens or hurts another. Effective anger management entails learned skills that we acquire through reading, one-on-one counseling or courses and skills groups that focus on anger management. Through anger management we learn three principles: to feel the anger, to own the anger, and to process the anger healthily.

The chronically challenged person needs to assume responsibility in this process and actively participate in the proper management of their anger. Misplaced anger or repressed anger is anger directed at another person or at oneself; both create unhealthy results. On the other hand, properly managed anger unclutters a person's emotional life and frees them from the heaviness of unprocessed anger. Anger management contributes to the person's holistic wellness.

Knowing and mastering effective communication techniques is something we learn; for most of us they are not natural skills. In order to communicate effectively, we must master the art of listening attentively as well as the art of speaking appropriately. The content of a conversation, the message I try to send is of equal value to the delivery, the way in which I send the message. When a chronically ill person tells her physician, "This incontinence bothers me and I want you to fix it," the physician will undoubtedly be turned off since the patient's request translates into an order. An alternate and effective message might be, "My incontinence is damaging my self-esteem and I am feeling overwhelmed by it; could you help me?" Notice the difference in the delivery style; a request from the speaker yields more than a demand ever does. *How* you say something is as important as *what* you say.

The caregiver who is not listening effectively may neglect to notice a decline in the ill person's morale. The body language signals or the verbal message, "I can't handle this anymore," may go unheard. Effective listening requires being attentive to body language and to indirect verbal communication. There exist many books, as well as many skilled professionals that can teach effective communication skills. Chronically challenged persons must express their thoughts, their feelings and their needs; only then will the channels open to holistic wellness.

Spiritual Wellness

For a person to be holistically well, they must also attend to the spiritual challenge they face. As presented in chapter five, if a person already has a relationship with a God of their own understanding, then maintenance and enhancement of this relationship with the soul comes easily. Often, the traumatic experience of chronic illness attacks our spiritual belief system which is shaken and then discarded. Just as often, with time and effective grieving, the basic value system and spiritual life does return. When chronic illness invades the life of someone who has not previously felt a need to develop a spiritual life, much grounding can come from a serious attempt to develop this dimension. Spiritual wellness brings a direction to our daily lives, a motivation to journey from day to day. A well soul focuses a person, whether they are chronically ill or not, toward holistic wellness.

Pictures provide paths toward a well state of soul and of mind. Mind images include pictures that we create from our own imagination; a chronically ill person can use these pictures as tools to visualize their own wellness. We need to always remember that wellness is not a *perfect* state of being, wellness is an *acceptable* state of being. Visualizing ourself as well physically, emotionally, and spiritually can be a powerful experience.

Our vizualization technique consists of setting the imagination free to take a mind picture. Next, the person, while comfortably at rest, will focus on this image. The more the mind avails itself of positive images and the more we have the chance to make regular use of these images, the less the chance of negative images or attitudes taking up valuable space in our lives. It takes a conscious decision to try visualization; it takes repetitive experimentation to reach a stage where we will reap the results of this exercise.

Meditation varies from visualization in that, although it taps into the mind, it utilizes our "speaking" thoughts. Actually we speak to ourself in our mind, or out loud if we choose. We select a brief written passage or a picture and engage in reflection and dialogue with ourself while focusing on the words or the image. We seek to reach the same objective: to fill our mind with constructive messages, with validating thoughts, something many of us do not receive enough of from others. Meditation as a daily activity yields marvellous results as the meditator moves closer and closer to soul wellness. Just as we maintain intimate communication with another person by speaking and listening to that person regularly, we maintain intimate communication with our inner life by engaging regularly in talking and listening to our soul.

Wellness for the Caregiver

In the same way that a chronically challenged person commits to working toward wellness, so the caregiver focuses on this same work: holistic wellness.

Focusing on the present is one of the greatest new challenges for the caregiver. As a caregiver, we fall into the trap of focusing on the future. The past is lost and the present seems dim. When we agonize over the future, the picture holds horrible images of more advanced stages of the illness that leave us more despairing than healthy. On the other hand, a caregiver who musters the strength to deal with chronic illness in a healthy way will transfer that same energy into the future. By focusing on living well *today* we guarantee that everything else will fall into place.

Many societies for chronic illnesses have established support groups for the caregivers; the realization that the family has the disease has come. No one really understands the experience of care giving until that experience is lived. These support networks offer attentive listening, a climate where each member can vent feelings about care giving.

Groups, however, don't suit everyone; the one-on-one aspect of counseling can be a viable option. Perhaps the society affiliated with the disease offers individual support; we do well to remember that the services are at our disposal and if not used, will cease to be. The caregiver may share with a friend or a family member, on a daily basis, whatever situations they find difficult to cope with. At intervals, the caregiver initiates a dialogue with the person he takes care of; often, the chronically challenged remains unaware of what the other role feels like. Whatever it takes to obtain support, we seek in order to provide the caregiver with a chance at holistic wellness.

Education plays a major role in assuring the wellness of the caregiver. At the onset of a chronic illness a caregiver must take time to gain all the knowledge possible about the disease. We gain the necessary information through libraries, medical offices, societies, or persons who have experienced the disease. This newfound knowledge will lessen the fear of the unknown, as well as create a boundary around what can be expected. Some people prefer not to know; in this case, they become targets for shocking fear or worse still, ill-informed about resources in terms of care. Holistic wellness demands that each person affected by the disease knows exactly what the other one faces.

Both the chronically challenged person and the caregiver must use effective communication. More than ever, the caregiver can suffer from isolation or feelings of being in a singular position. Only another person can mirror that experience. By communicating effectively with the patient, the caregiver diffuses his own feelings about the situation.

Emotional breakdown plagues caregivers; people just snap under the emotional weight of care giving, usually because they have not cared sufficiently for themselves. Communication treats and assures proper self-care. The need to verbalize and the need to be heard make up the basic neccesities in communication. An invitation to the chronically ill person is appropriate and allows the caregiver to check out the patient's desire to talk about good or bad news.

In some cases it might be advisable for both the challenged partner and the caregiver to meet with a professional counselor. Communicating effectively will not take away the pain of the situation; it will, however, lessen its impact and lead to wellness for the caregiver.

Should I bring the challenged person a glass of water, or should I suggest they get it? This is the dilemma of responsibility. Ideally, the chronically ill person needs to assume their responsibility as much as possible; this creates for them a healthy self-image and a sense of control over their own life. The caregiver should tune in to the degree of ability that the challenged person has to meet their own needs. At all times, promoting responsiblity on the part of the ill person is preferable. It is appropriate of course to assist the challenged person and satisfy their needs if they cannot accomplish it themselves.

One universal law applies to this patient/caregiver partnership*: as a caregiver, you cannot fix it!* The caregiver assumes no responsibility for the disease, for its progression nor for its outcome. Always, the chronically challenged person signs the contract, willing or not, as the ultimate author of their life; they agree to live with the predetermined condition. Effective communication illuminates the way so that the caregiver and their support network can journey toward the same goal.

Being a caregiver to someone with multiple sclerosis, for example, means living with multiple sclerosis; you may not have it, but you live with it. The challenge for the caregiver can be as great as that for the ill person. The holistic approach to wellness is crucial to a quality of life.

When lived well, care giving becomes a most rewarding experience. This demanding experience requires some emotional and spiritual stretching. Time provides skills and knowledge. Effective communication can be permanently established with time and practice. Care giving, which is a precious gift, offers a magnificent view into the world of the chronically challenged person.

Husband Sues to Spend Night A Week with Paralyzed Wife

By Sonia Barisic
ASSOCIATED PRESS

CINCINNATI–Barry Belinky says he only wanted to spend one night a week cuddling with his wife of 31 years.

But [the] long term care hospital where she lives, paralyzed and barely able to speak, refused. It fears that if the couple have sex, it could be considered rape because Diane Belinky cannot give her consent.

So Belinky sued.

His lawsuit was to have gone to trial yesterday but Judge Robert Ruehlman dismissed the case Tuesday without explanation.

Belinky, 53, who insists he has no intention of having sex with his wife, said he will appeal.

"She's confused and scared, and it was my opinion that...it would be helpful for me to be able to stay over," he said in an interview from his home in Finneytown, a Cincinnati suburb. The Belinkys have two daughters, 25 and 23.

Diane, a 54-year-old synagogue administrator was admitted to the Drake Centre in 1994 after an aneurysm in her brain ruptured.

The couple's marriage therapist wrote to the hospital recommending Belinky be allowed to spend the night in his wife's bed.

In a memo to the therapist, Shearer, Drake's vice-president of nursing, indicated the request was rejected because of the possibility the couple might have sex.

"Case law in this area is very clear; any type of sexual relations in the absence of consent is rape," Shearer wrote.

That, in turn, could open the hospital to a lawsuit.

Hospital spokesperson Kay Nolen also said Belinky's presence after visiting hours could violate other patient's privacy, disrupt the staff and create a safety hazard.

"We're not running a hotel. We're running a health-care facility," she said yesterday.

After Belinky sued, the hospital in October began allowing him to spend one night a week with his wife pending the outcome of the case.

Diane can speak, but most of her words are unintelligible, Belinky's lawyer William Knapp said. She cannot use her legs or left arm and is at times unresponsive. Doctors have given her husband no hope her condition will improve.

Belinky, a chemist, said it was a nurse at the hospital who first suggested he ask permission to spend the night with his wife.

"When I do stay here, I essentially don't get any sleep at all," he said. His wife must be turned over every two hours so she doesn't get bed sores.

"When they come in, I have to get out of the bed," he said. When they're done, I stroke her head until she goes to sleep."

The Case of Diane Belinky

The Diane Belinky case raises controversial questions on the subject of holistic wellness. Among the ethical, medical and political questions are:

Would precedence be set in the event that the husband were allowed to spend nights with his wife in the hospital?

How could medical health professionals attend to Diane differently?

What about the patient's choices?

What constitutes the rights of the caregiver (in this case, the husband)?

The husband's motive translates into nonsexual affection for his wife; both he and their marriage therapist had concluded that spending the night would help alleviate some of Diane's anxieties. Granted, in its uniqueness, this situation presents newness and a possible change of routine for the nursing staff. Although we agree that a health-care facility is not a hotel, we must keep in mind that Diane is not on a holiday; she and her husband would never choose this facility if they were looking for a romantic evening. Night often triggers the worst time for chronically ill persons; out come all of the emotional bogey men and the insomnia sweats. It would appear that Barry has done his homework; clearly, his objective – to comfort her, "to stroke her hair" while she is confused and fearful – warrants respect. We hope the courts in this case would decide in favor of holistic wellness even if that meant a disruption for the medical facility. There *are* some individuals with the power to make changes who value the holistic approach as an obligatory necessity for the chronically challenged. Those in power situations who have not yet realized the impact of holistic wellness continue to operate low-quality care facilities which have so much potential to be transformed into "wholly" healing facilities.

The Ultimate Declaration of Wellness

ואהבת את הוה אלהך בכל לבבך ובפל

Love the Lord your God with all your heart, with all your soul, with all your means. Deuteronomy. 6:5-9

The first line of the Shema, the ultimate Hebrew prayer, declares the major tenet of the Judaic faith. This prayer, intended to be recited to God, views God as the perfect "whole" and "well" existence. Moreover, it stipulates that we are created in that image of God, therefore, *we are created holistically well.* Notice the three dimensions of the human being: the heart, the soul and the means. These refer to the triad of the emotional, the spiritual and the physical dimensions of a person. We function wholly when all three aspects work together toward a total wellness. A conscious decision to pursue wellness and unrelenting efforts to maintain that wellness assures quality of life. We are never alone, except by choice.

Our commonality as human beings helps us actively participate in our wellness. We have our entire life cycles in common: from childhood programming, to adolescent crises, to career goal setting, not to mention gender related issues and everyday life challenges. We can glean from this commonality, much emotional and psychological energy for "whole"istic wellness.

The expression "Been there, done that," carries with it the implication that others have "been there" before you, that "You are not alone." How have others begun their journeys toward wellness? Which steps did they take as they charted their course toward wellness? How do they maintain their wellness? We are intended in our commonality to act as mirrors for each other. The more effectively we use our mirrors, the more effectively we will achieve and maintain our own holistic wellness.

EIGHT

Heroes and Heroines

The Professional Dancers

My Champions

Their illness speaks my language
Their passion speaks my call
Their faith speaks motivation and hope
In the strength of us all.

From their lifeless legs, I walk up my Masada
With their glassy eyes, I see my inner being
In their depressed souls, I am gifted with solace
From their courage, I am infused with hope.

Their cancer teaches me the quality of life
Their blindness paints a mosaic of veritable insight
Their wheelchairs transport me on uncharted highways
Their minds teach me wisdom.

I am blind
I am crippled
I am depressed
I am dying
I dance with the professional dancers.

We learn to dance with chronic illness with its physical, emotional or mental challenges in order to live fully. Among the various management aids we can acquire, the adoption of a "Champions" list – heroes who have similar challenges, who have succeeded or presently triumph over challenges – can give us inspiration.

When I noticed my son's collection of sports cards displaying his heroes, I began to draw up my own collection of heroes. Those with chronic illness, without sight, hearing, legs, mobility, or long-term peace of mind, had more insight, more voice and more quality of life in some cases than other persons I knew in the "abled" circle. My new life with chronic illness compelled me to pay attention to the challenged people already in my life. Isolation often accompanies challenge; I was lonely and robbed of my identity. My champions proved that I could not only survive, but develop a new life, abundant with quality and fulfilment. I was no longer alone; I joined the club of the "exceptional professional dancers."

How have I come to choose my champions? For the most part, the energy produced from being in their presence played the major role in my decision. Somehow after speaking or being with them, I experienced a sense of empowerment. Their challenges figure among the common diseases of our modern times: cancer, AIDS, multiple sclerosis. From ordinary roots, through ordinary paths, my champions share with the Olympians the sweet celebration of victory over adversity and suffering. In effect, I seek courage from *ordinary* people who have mastered the dance with chronic illness.

On the following pages, each champion's card presents the following information:

name of champion
year of birth (and death in some cases)
challenge
quote from the champion
gift from the champion to the world.

The Ballerina

Sylvie Bourré

1974 – 1991

CANCER

"There is nothing to fear in death."

BEAUTY

I remember the first time Sylvie came into my guidance office. I said, "Of course," to her request to sit in my chair because she wanted to play my role. The short time I spent with her touched me in places I had never known before. Sylvie Bourré was diagnosed with cancer five years before her death. After being given six months to live, she celebrated four more birthdays. She was 17 when she died.

"Have you lost more weight?" She interrogated me each day. "Well, chips for you Madame." The routine consisted of her delivering munchies each morning as she paid her regular visit to my office. Sylvie sported different caps while her hair thinned and disappeared. Her gorgeous sculptured nails and her impish allure added to a wisdom and insight that reached far beyond her years.

We became friends, so when I had my own battle to fight against multiple sclerosis, we made contact, each from our respective medical clinics. She was trying desperately to accept her chemotherapy while I was desperately trying to work at my physiotherapy. With a quivering voice, Sylvie, now as fragile as I had ever known her to be, managed to say, "Hold on, don't hang up," while her body shook and she vomited the horrendous effects of chemotherapy. Even if we spoke little on that memorable day, I sensed the Herculean strength of that delicate bird over the telephone wire. I was made stronger myself through her.

Sylvie studied intensely to catch up with all the days she missed while in treatment. She walked with a bounce while she giggled with her friends. She challenged the teachers who objected to her nibbling and drinking in class to settle her weak ravaged stomach.

She spoke to me of death, of her own death, not removed, but more like the author of that inevitable passage. "I figure, if you believe in God, then dying has to be better than living. Besides, I can't wait to see my mom and dad."

I replied, "Are you afraid of dying, Sylvie?"

"Not really...the next chemo week, that's scary!"

Not once did I hear rage from her lips; the mild sadness that sometimes came over her was perfectly tender. Sylvie spoke often of being with her parents, who were deceased, as she adhered to a religious devotion that she never lost.

As I entered the funeral parlor, my legs shook and I began to sob; to witness this beautiful child/woman lying so still in a casket was almost too much for me to bear. "She is a sleeping beauty," I whispered to my husband. A sleeping beauty, a sleeping ballerina who has gifted the world and especially those she came in contact with. I recognized the strength and the courage of this inspirational champion.

The high school where she attended awards a plaque every year in the memory of Sylvie Bourré, an honor bestowed upon someone with outstanding courage. Those who receive it are taught all about the delicate girl with the awesome power.

The Positive Dancer

Melvin Chelsky
1939 –
BLINDNESS

"I would never take back my sight if it meant losing my insight."

POSITIVISM

He arrived by airplane. I had asked a committee person to pick him up since our telephone call had left me thinking he was arrogant and full of himself. Five years later, I married him.

Melvin Chelsky was born with congenital cataracts on both eyes. When he was a toddler, his brother, who was then in medical school, noticed the baby's awkwardness and concluded that little Melvin was blind. At the age of three, the eye surgeries began. He struggled under the famous ether mask and endured seemingly endless stays in hospital wards, strapped to beds. A few years after many such operations, Melvin, for the first time in his life, could see relatively well, with one of his eyes.

He was sent to a school for mentally and emotionally challenged children. That year was a nightmare since the other kids stole his lunches and called him all sorts of names because of his awkwardness and his thick glasses. Finally, his parents realized their error and enrolled him in regular classes. He proved to be a whiz, in no time catching up academically to his peers.

No one believed that he would amount to much, people even said that they would eat their hats if he ever graduated from anything. Melvin's determination led him on to an apprenticeship with an accountant; at the age of 25 he became a Chartered Accountant. His career brought him to government positions, to industry, and ultimately to private practice.

At the age of 36 in the space of one day, his "good" eye hemorrhaged; the diagnosis: detached retina. Melvin was left legally blind. Like other "low vision" people, the way he maneuvers around makes it difficult to believe the legal blindness. Most persons cannot believe that he is blind; he has adopted none of the traditional mannerisms. Only when you share a home with him do you realize all the toe-stubbing, the head-banging into cupboard doors, and the searching for things that goes on. His toes have all been broken at one time or another as testimonial that he can't see where he's going.

Melvin Chelsky shines as a truly exceptional human being who happens to be blind; there is no focus on his disability, only a true sense of positivism and humor for the limitations that he has. One time when I complained about having to drive with hand-controls, he added that it was better than having two seeing-eye dogs dragging my car. He lives life to the fullest, travels extensively, gets the groceries. He reads the newspaper by deciphering one syllable at a time, moving his head back and forth across the page, which he holds about one inch from his face. He takes his dog for walks and watches baseball and Letterman. All the many things he does to make life "un-disabled," challenging and fulfilling, make up the hero that he is.

The Angel

Betty Cummings

1923 – 1996

STROKE/CANCER

"Nice."

ANGELIC STRENGTH

As soon as the IV was hooked up to me, the treatment began its roaring fire into my veins; it would save my eyes, it had to. Since the curtain was drawn, the only evidence of my roommate, whom I had not yet seen, was the periodic uttering of the word, "nice." Whenever a nurse would attend to her, I would hear those "nice" words, followed by the attendant's praise for "Betty," who seemingly was quite a charmer.

Once the treatment was over for that first day, I ventured from my bed to scout around my room, this domain, this prison where I would live profound experiences within the next few days. It was no Hilton, but it was satisfactory for the task.

When Betty saw me, her face lit up and I sensed her genuine struggle to say hello; alas, no words were uttered and I quickly surmised that she could not speak. Her right hand motioned "hello" to me while her left hand and arm lay lifeless alongside her body. After my "Hi there roomy, I'm Louise," I received the gift of my first "Nice," which meant everything. The next day, when I helped her with her juice, she said, "Louise," followed by an ecstasy from her voice that seemed to say, "I've practiced all night to say this to you, you'd better appreciate it."

During the night I heard her stirring and almost moaning only to find her frozen. She had buzzed but the staff was so hecticly busy that no one had come to cover her. As I cuddled Betty with all the blankets I could find, I bent down and stroked her forehead; she touched my cheek with her good hand and said, "Nice." That's when I fell in love with Betty Cummings. Only with time would I come to realize just how powerful she would be in my life.

In the mornings, our husbands came in with fresh coffee for their girls; Frank and Melvin became immediate buddies. Both talked endlessly about their "working" years in accounting and in the police force. Many humorous times were had while they read their newspapers and watched their princesses sleep. When Frank teased Betty, she would manage to utter, "Stop, Frank," which meant, "Never stop teasing and loving me, Frank."

Betty had worked as a physiotherapist for over 30 years at the same hospital. She had been chairperson of the Physiotherapists Association and on every committee one could dream of. Soon after her retirement at the age of 57, she suffered a stroke which left her paralyzed on one side; there never was much recovery. She was hospitalized at least 20 times in eight years and suffered from Paget's disease, a rare form of bone cancer. The hospital knew of her reputation as an angel of strength and if the staff could have bid on who would attend to her, they would have.

A few months after our initial meeting, I was "out" and she was "in." Since Melvin had nicknamed her Betty Boop, we brought over a pink nightshirt with the caricature, the huge eyeballs and overdone eyelashes. Betty summoned someone to put her into her shirt and the only time it left her was for washing. After many months of hospitalization, she was given respite in her home, where I would take my dog to visit with her. Bart licked her paralyzed hand while the smile on her face lit up the room. He sat glued to the carpet beside her and slowly the same hand gathered the strength to stroke his head. The communication between them was phenomenal.

At the end of the ravages of a cold winter, Betty died peacefully. As she came in and out of consciousness, she kissed Frank good-bye, dying in the arms of the man she loved so much. My pain was profound, I could hardly bring myself to weep. I was forgetting that Betty had been promoted to "angel." The realization came the day when I received her wheelchair as my own. I ride the wheelchair of a champion: her name is Betty Cummings. I am supported and empowered by my chair, the chair of a champion. I ride on an angel's wings.

The Dance of Hope

Norm Fera
1954 – 1994
Multiple Sclerosis

**"Never give up...
always hope."**

HOPE

The first time I met Norm Fera, we did exercises on a mat during a Yoga class for persons with multiple sclerosis. Norm had been diagnosed ten years previously; he now resided in the chronic ward of the same hospital. My first reaction was to take care of him: after all wasn't he in far worse shape than I? He immediately made it clear that he did not need caretaking from me. I was inspired by this champion and recognized his courage and optimism. Norm would never be beaten, I thought. Everyone who knew him soon came to the same conclusion. Norm always spoke of the Mighty Strange disease that afflicted us, about the hope for a cure, about how we had to keep fighting.

Little by little, over the next few years, my encounters with him were more and more painful for me as I watched MS rob him of his sight, his speech, his respiration, his whole physical capacity. Not once did I witness visible desperation or gloom from him; on the contrary, every meeting with him left me with a sadness for his losses, a rage for the ravages of the disease, and a new energy to live my life to the fullest in spite of multiple sclerosis.

In the course of the last few years of his life, Norm fought on with miraculous strength. When the physicians rendered a sentence of impending death, Norm would come back as a giant phoenix. After 14 years of battle, the Beast MS finally sucked all physical life from Norm Fera and he died peacefully.

Many of us with multiple sclerosis who knew Norm Fera hold his courage very much alive in our hearts and in our minds. The memory of his unwavering smile is a constant reminder of the potential in all of us to fight, to win the war, to never give up hope.

The Waltzer

Paul Giroux
1910 – 1977
MULTIPLE SCLEROSIS

"Never complain about being busy... it's idle time that is sufferance."

FAITH

At the age of 40, Paul was labeled "terminal" and given 3 months to live. Three months later, he sat in his hospital bed and smiled for the camera in order to send a photo to his kids for Christmas. For 27 years following his primary diagnosis, Paul lived with multiple sclerosis. With his courage and especially with profound faith in the God of his understanding, the would-be "terminal" patient made an amazing recovery from his initial physical paralysis.

His sense of humor was always sharp, even during the bouts of exacerbating multiple sclerosis. His wisdom became more and more noticeable as he took his idle time to reflect on life and its meaning. The days dragged by while everyone in the family attended to their responsibilities. Paul, an illiterate, spent those longs days in thought and in prayer. At lunchtime, his children would warm up with the hot tomato rice soup their father had cooked up. From his permanent seat in his chair, Paul cooked, did laundry, practiced woodworking.

During the course of his life with multiple sclerosis, Paul became a caregiver to his wife who fought a war against cancer and finally died at the age of 49. He would take soup upstairs to her by dragging himself along the floor and up the steps. Throughout these few years, he was her source of courage and hope. Whenever she asked how he managed to take over this way, his response was, "You taught me well, Florence."

When his wife died, only their baby was left at home to care for him. I was 13; some concerned persons wanted to take charge of my care. We were brought before a judge who would rule on the situation. My father, from his wheelchair, stated, "I always thought that raising a child had to do with having a brain and having a heart; the fact that I don't have use of my legs has nothing to do with it." The judge dismissed the request and told both of us to go home.

His creative mind sought out ways to bring resource people into my life, to fill the gap with the things he could not provide. Many years after he befriended a young woman, I figured out the role model he had chosen for me. When he concerned himself with my school results, he called my teachers and spent long conversations with them until he made sense of the academic jargon.

When I started high school, I showed an interest in writing. "Here is your tool to write," was all he said when a store clerk delivered my first typewriter. I wondered where Paul got the money to pay for this tool. Years later he shared that, for five years, he put aside the cost of a package of tobacco every week, so that he could accumulate the $139 for the Underwood typewriter. Although his disease consumed a great part of his energy, he managed to parent effectively, because he took his responsibility seriously.

Paul Giroux believed in the power of prayer. He lost every one of his bodily functions to multiple sclerosis, but he never lost his faith. In the midst of poverty, of geographical isolation, and of personal physical suffering, his giant spirit left strength as a legacy to his family and to all those afflicted with chronic illness.

Dance of Serenity

Kenneth Hodges
1925 – 1994
CANCER

**"I'm not so special.
We all have the strength
to fight cancer."**

SERENITY

As I glanced outside my kitchen window, I noticed Ken watering his flowers; his hair was now starting to grow back. His care for each one of these precious and delicate flowers elevated him as a man dedicated to tenderness. I celebrated the regrowth of his hair since he had talked about the ordeal of losing it. This was an opportunity for me to go out and talk with him and to welcome him back after his ordeal with chemotherapy. Ken Hodges had been diagnosed with cancer a few years before his death; against all odds, he maintained a good quality of life until the very end.

Once I remarked, "You are exceptional; you inspire me." He responded, "No, I am ordinary; you would be the same way. We all do what we have to do." I was not convinced of that since I had and have seen since, people who are afflicted and not coping exceptionally well with their challenge. Ken read Bernie Siegel, went to his granddaughter's riding competitions, his grandson's hockey games and out every morning for his newspaper. Just a month before his death, Ken found the strength to fight the dandelions on his lawn and to manicure his cedar hedges.

Each time I would speak with him, he always shared his concern for me: How was I doing with my illness? Ken had the ability to look away from his own suffering in order to care for others. After each chemo treatment, he would regain his pride in his new hair and enjoy each waking moment like never before.

I spent some time with him in his hospital room the few days before his death. Every so often he would wake up, only to say, "You should go home and get some rest." Ken did not focus on his condition which he knew only too well, but rather extended his concern to his caregivers.

His selfless death leaves us with a lesson in coping with chronic illness; it must never become a focal point but rather always remain an underlying condition to a perfectly healthy state of mind and state of heart. Wellness of our mind encompasses serenity and acceptance of the challenge. Wellness of heart emits love to others, a love always going away from us towards others.

The Up-Beat Dancer

Nathan Klegerman

1929 – 1991

EMPHYSEMA/CANCER

"Study is for your mind the first order of business."

SELF-DISCIPLINE

As I walked into his room, I knew all too well that this would be the last time I saw him. Nathan lay, a fragile shell of what he used to be, journeying into the corridor between life and death. I touched his white hair and thanked him for all he had brought to my life in the five years I had known him. And I sobbed. Nathan Klegerman died a few days later.

Bullus emphysema, a respiratory disease, plagued him with pneumothoraxes, attacks when his lungs collapsed and he could not breath. Eleven years after the onset of his chronic disease, he was diagnosed with colon cancer. During the first years of his challenge with respiratory disease, Nathan underwent stringent rehabilitation for over nine months. He needed to learn to maximize his breathing strategies, something most of us take for granted as a normal, basic function. He developed a state-of-the-art mastery of his breathing; many professionals in the medical community of respiratory illness coined him a Master Breather.

But it was not only for his physical mastery of breathing that I call him a champion. Nathan had a brilliant mind and a profound positive emotional life. That combination would make his many years of living with chronic illness fulfilled years, with an abundance of quality of life. Many times during each day, he read and studied the Jewish Scriptures, his source of wisdom and courage. Many people came to him for advice about living, about relationships, about everything. Somehow, he remained capable of using everything he learned and of applying the knowledge to everyday living.

Having studied philosophy, Nathan continued to be a thinker; his interests turned to theology as well. On his bedside table were stacked many books, all of which were laden with napkins or tissues, his reference spots for further thought processing. Each day carried with it an opportunity to learn, to debate, to think and to pray.

With his family, Nathan perpetuated a strong sense of effective relationships. He treasured his grandsons, taught his son about life, cajoled his daughter, and admired his partner. Always his attention went outward to his loved ones, a character trait that made him charming and deeply respected by all who knew him.

He was motivated to live with a healthy intellect, to remain positive and upbeat no matter which adversity came. Above all, his concern for others touched so many. Today, when my mind wanders back to the final good-bye at his bedside, I do not see a fragile shell of a man, but a giant among champions.

The Little Prince

Richard Robert Leroux
1962 – 1996
AIDS

"Suffering is being without love."

SPIRITUAL ENERGY

"I can't let him go!" I muttered through my sobs. Something told me that I would never see Richard alive again. It was a selfish sob, a sob for me; each moment spent with him enriched me, empowered me, gave me courage beyond my expectations. All this from a dying man.

Richard Robert Leroux was 13 when I taught him in grade eight. By his questions, his curiosity, and his animated personality, I knew that this little boy would be somebody special. His artistic nature screamed to be set free; it took its wings with every research project that I assigned. More than most of the others in the class, his humorous responses and intelligent inquisitions made him a favorite for me. That year, his father died suddenly at the age of 39. Wise beyond his years, Richard grasped the symbolic meaning of the quote, "The essential is invisible to the eyes," written by St. Exupéry in *The Little Prince.* I presented him with a rose at his father's funeral and we became kindred spirits.

Twenty-one years later, I presented him with three roses: mind, heart, and body. Richard was now 34, and dying of AIDS. As I approached him, he had risen from his bed, all piped-up, but amazingly looking much the very same as he did when he was 13, with that impish grin, those curious eyes seeking knowledge. I could not deny the visible signs of his impending death: the leg colored by melanoma, the greenish hue of his skin, the sores on his chest. However, from that moment on, I became imbued with a strength that was addictive; his strength hooked me. "I am dying, the welcome mat to Death is laid out for me." I shook at the openness, the candor, the stability of his voice. "I know exactly where I am going." I was dumbfounded yet so curious. "No, I am not afraid. This is my preparation time."

Pills of every color and size were strewn all over his home, "La ville" as he called it. I handed him a thimble of morphine which he downed immediately. The IV in his arm dripped slowly, supposedly relieving some of the migraine caused by his meningitis. As he vomited violently, I stroked his back and my tears welled up. When he sat down again, I commented, "You are suffering, it hurts me to see you suffering."

"No, this is not suffering. Suffering is not being with physical pain or without food. Suffering is being without love. I have love all around me. I am not suffering."

Silence followed. In that silence, the thundering truth came to me; I was in the presence of a unique man, a powerhouse of wisdom. I could not tear myself away from him.

The teacher became the pupil. Richard taught me how to live with chronic illness and suffering. I listened and learned. I asked and he answered. He asked to move into the garden, his garden, planted and nurtured by him. With the assistance of his nurse, we managed to transform a patio chair into a bed and his fragile body rested. As he dozed off for a while, I sat and watched him. This is what suffering is all about; seizing the opportunity to become more. Going through the death passage, savoring every moment of the journey, walking acceptingly to the other side. There is a purpose to it all.

Reverberating in my ears are the words of St. Exupéry: "The essential is invisible to the eyes." I sit with my Little Prince, Richard, breathing in his exceptional energy, listening to his pearls of wisdom, laughing at his poignant comments. How small and in need of learning I am myself next to this giant among my champions.

Who wears the title of professional dancer? An ordinary two-stepping person transformed into a master dancer. What does it take to become a professional dancer? A dream and persistence.

We choose to pursue our dream or to let it die, whether we are chronically challenged or not. Why does a dream have to end with the birth of disease? Can we alter the same dream to fit the new challenge? Even when we have to choose another dream, as long as we keep a dream alive, we will find the energy to sustain us in our attainment of that dream.

Persistence is courage; and courage is fear having said its prayers. When we hit rough spots in the road, we go around them, we detour. We climb one step at a time, to the top. We persevere, always keeping our sights on our dream.

The professional, chronically challenged persons included in my catalogue of champions are members of an Olympic team; they discovered deep within themselves the courage to fight. That same courage exists for all of us. Courage weaves the fabric of our essence, of who we are, and the vitality of life within ourselves – our soul.

We let our champions inspire us, encourage us, carry us. If they could be gold medal winners, professional dancers, why not us?

CONCLUSION

I'd Love To Dance

Either I learned to dance with my chronic illness, or
I would die under the weight of my chronic illness. I chose to live.

Learning is not easy. I have had to forget some preconceived notions, imagine some new notions and accept other notions from new teachers. At 36, I was ill prepared to start learning to live again differently. Like most of us, my road map was a clear road to productive success. I discovered that there is more than one road to a destination. How naive I was prior to getting my chronic illness. Stuck in the tornado of a profession where there was never time to stop, to think and to be.

At first my awkwardness in dancing with chronic illness was noticeable. I became "Ms. MS" in my area; every piece of literature was studied and spewed out again for all who would listen. The colossal fear of getting in touch with the Beast itself, the illness, overwhelmed me. Not until my rage grew to gigantic proportions did I succumb to face the Beast. Ever so slowly, I discovered that I could influence this disease. Perhaps it held the upper hand in the physical part of who I was, but it had no character, no spirit, no intellect. I realized that I was in charge after all. By calming it, by letting it have its own way once in a while, the Beast became a tamed dance partner.

When my optic neuritis attacked my eyes, I learned to let them rest. When my hands began to tremble, I rested my body. If my short-term memory failed me, I used Post-it notes. Catheterizing alleviated the problem of residual fluids in my bladder and bulk foods became the solution to my bowel dysfunction. I met other challenged persons who were giants of the spiritual world and I allowed myself to be influenced by them. My own way of coping with my Beast began to emerge and the more I led the dance the more I believed that I was in command.

Often, within the imaging of a meditation, I am dancing a ballroom waltz; in a flowing satin gown, a minute body leads the Giant Beast towering over me. It is as though the Beast actually respects me. To the melody of a unique chorus, we dance. The music of my soul fills the air as *I dance with my Chronic Illness.*

RECOMMENDED READINGS

1. Barasch, Marc Ian. (1983). *The Healing Path.* New York, Penguin Books.

2. Cleveland, Martha. (1989). *Living Well.* San Francisco, Harper & Row Publishers.

3. Coffey-Lewis, Lou. (1984). *Be Restored to Health.* Toronto, Random House of Canada.

4. Cousins, Norman. (1989). *Head First: the Biology of Hope.* Toronto, E.P. Dutton.

5. Giroux, Louise. (1997). *Healing Times: A Personal Workbook.* Kelowna, Northstone Publishing.

6. – (1995). *Recycled: A Story of Hope.* Toronto, Fenix Ryzing Associates.

7. Frankl, Viktor. (1986). *The Doctor and the Soul.* New York, Vintage Books.

8. Hay, Louise. (1984). *You Can Heal Your Life.* CA, Hay House.

9. LeMaistre, JoAnn. (1985). *Beyond Rage.* Illinois, Alpine Guild.

10. McKay, Rogers & McKay. (1989). *When Anger Hurts.* CA, New Harbinger Publications.

11. Siegel, Bernie. (1986). *Love, Medicine and Miracles.* NY, Harper and Row Publishers.

12. – (1990). *Peace, Love and Healing.* NY, Harper and Row Publishers.

13. – (1993). *How to Live Between Office Visits.* NY, HarperCollins Publishers.